Study Guide for

Pathophysiology

Study Guide

Jacquelyn L. Banasik

Pathophysiology

Sixth Edition

Prepared by:
Jacquelyn L. Banasik, PhD, ARNP
Associate Professor
College of Nursing
Washington State University
Spokane, Washington

ELSEVIER

ELSEVIER

3251 Riverport Lane
St. Louis, Missouri 63043

STUDY GUIDE FOR PATHOPHYSIOLOGY, SIXTH EDITION ISBN: 978-0-3234-4429-3

Notices

Executive Content Strategist: Kellie White
Senior Content Development Manager: Luke Held
Content Development Specialist: Jennifer Wade
Publishing Services Manager: Deepthi Unni
Project Manager: Radhika Sivalingam
Cover Designer: Muthukumaran Thangaraj

Printed in the United States of America

Last digit is the print number: 9 8 7 6 5 4 3 2 1

Working together
to grow libraries in
developing countries

www.elsevier.com • www.bookaid.org

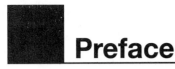

Preface

Pathophysiology is a complex and ever-expanding subject. In an effort to provide students with a comprehensive reference, *pathophysiology* texts contain a large amount of information, facts, and details. The Banasik & Copstead text, *Pathophysiology,* sixth edition, includes Key Questions and Key Points to help the student focus on the important concepts. This workbook builds on that approach by providing Practice Questions that correspond to the ideas presented in each chapter of the textbook and Case Studies at the end of each unit. Many students of pathophysiology are uncertain about the adequacy of their knowledge, even after they have read and studied, particularly as examination time draws near. This student study guide is designed to focus on the important concepts and to help students build confidence in their knowledge base and test-taking skills.

Although this workbook follows the organization of the Banasik & Copstead textbook, it can also be used in the context of other courses or as a refresher before taking the NCLEX® examination.

I hope you find it useful.

Jacquelyn L. Banasik

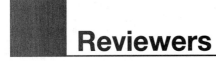

Reviewers

Amber Ballard MSN, RN
Sparrow Health System, Michigan State University
Home Care; Learning and Assessment Center
Lansing, Michigan

Keys to Success

The amount of information contained in a typical pathophysiology text can be daunting, but a number of strategies are available to help students grasp the underlying concepts and therefore be able to retain the information and apply it. For many students, nursing school provides at least one educational challenge they have not experienced previously—the need to apply knowledge learned in various theory classes to their patients in the clinical setting. Relying on old techniques of memorizing for examinations and then moving on to the next topic will no longer work. Your theory classes may not have comprehensive examinations, but your clinical practice will surely require that previous knowledge be retained and applied in a variety of situations. This is not to say that you will not need to memorize some things; rather, you will need to know why you are memorizing and how these memorized facts fit into concepts that will help you sort out assessment findings in clinical practice situations.

Keep Your Purpose in Mind

Before setting out to study pathophysiology, thinking about the purpose for knowing this information will help you focus on the main points. Nurses use pathophysiology for three main purposes:

1. *To predict the clinical manifestations likely to be present in a patient with a known medical diagnosis.* Predicting the clinical manifestations allows the nurse to tailor the assessment of the patient and to monitor the signs and symptoms that indicate whether the patient is improving or getting worse. Assessment findings that do not seem to fit with the patient's diagnosis can also be recognized and investigated.
2. *To formulate hypotheses about the meaning of clinical findings and their causes.* Each pathophysiologic process has characteristic or typical manifestations that usually accompany it. One finding is seldom enough to lead to a diagnosis; rather, a constellation of findings indicates a problem. Manifestations often vary from person to person, making the detective work more difficult. Because of their close contact with patients, nurses are often the first to suspect a pathologic problem in a patient. A good understanding of pathophysiologic processes allows for early recognition and the initiation of therapy. For example, the findings of fever, increased respiratory rate, shallow breathing, and adventitious breath sounds in a patient after a surgical procedure may indicate the development of hypostatic pneumonia. An astute nurse can intervene early and reduce morbidity.
3. *To evaluate the appropriateness of prescribed therapies and assess for possible contraindications.* The pathophysiologic mechanisms of particular disease processes usually imply which treatment may be effective and which may be contraindicated. For example, a patient with coronary heart disease may be appropriately prescribed a β-adrenergic–blocking drug to reduce cardiac workload; however, if the patient also has low blood pressure, then the drug may exacerbate the hypotension. This situation requires that the blood pressure be monitored closely and that the person responsible for writing the prescription be made aware of the problem.

Thus, asking yourself how the information you are reading in the text will be applied clinically will be helpful. This technique will keep you focused on the important points and also provide the motivation for learning the material; a patient will be depending on your knowledge base. Few things are more satisfying in clinical practice than diagnosing a problem early and preventing a patient from experiencing serious consequences. In this regard, the application of pathophysiology is a rewarding kind of detective work—and it is fun to solve the case!

Apply Pathophysiology to Life

Pathophysiology is everywhere! Conversations with your next-door neighbor, complaints from your family members, and medical dramas on television provide good practice in honing your assessment and diagnostic skills. Try to analyze the signs you observe, and predict a diagnosis—before the television episode reveals the answer. (Do not, however, dispense your medical opinion. That will get you into big trouble. This is simply an exercise of the mind.)

When you begin your first clinical rotation, you will have opportunities to apply your knowledge to real situations. Although focusing on tasks and learning to communicate with patients are natural, be sure to spend some focused time trying to understand your patient's pathophysiology. Look up the laboratory findings. Note the physical signs and symptoms. Try to correlate these with the medical diagnosis. Look over the medications to determine whether they make sense with regard to the diagnosis. Ask your clinical instructor questions when you are not sure. (Do not be afraid of showing your ignorance. Clinical instructors generally appreciate a curious student!) Take every available opportunity to apply the concepts you are learning in your pathophysiology course.

ix

Know the Relevant Anatomy and Physiology

Students who have a good grasp of anatomy and physiology (A&P) tend to have an easier time understanding pathophysiology. Conversely, students who are no longer facile with A&P are likely to struggle and find that they must review the normal structures and functions before they can proceed. The Banasik & Copstead textbook incorporates such reviews into each unit. The best place to start learning pathophysiology is to get A&P into your working knowledge. In this study guide, questions applicable to these review chapters are also provided. If answering these questions does not come easy, then you will benefit from reading the physiology review chapter in the text. The importance of a good basis in A&P cannot be overemphasized!

Develop Good Study Skills

Depending on your learning style, you may find one or more of the following general study tips to be helpful:

- Read with a purpose. Use the Key Questions to help focus on the major concepts as you read. Use the Key Points sections in each chapter to review what you have read and to test your understanding.
- Pay attention to new words. Vocabulary is a major part of learning new content; pathophysiology has its own language, and you need to learn it. A glossary at the back of the textbook is provided to help you.
- Memorize what you must, such as the normal values for arterial blood gases. However, think through the application to ensure that you understand it. (Why does pH go down when Pco_2 goes up?)
- Put facts into patterns. Sometimes, the patterns are obvious; other times, you have to create them. Mnemonics are helpful to remember some things, such as the order of the cranial nerves.
- Put what you have read into your own words. If you can explain a concept to someone else so that he or she understands it, then you know you really understand it yourself!
- Do not forget that pathophysiology predicts presentation. When you believe you understand the pathophysiology, make a list of the likely signs and symptoms that the abnormality suggests. Then go back and check your thinking. Being able to figure out the clinical manifestations as predicted by the underlying mechanisms is better than memorizing them.
- Recognize how you learn best. Some people learn best by reading information. Others find listening is better for them, and reading aloud and listening to tape recordings of classes is best. Some people make drawings or "trees" that show the relationships of ideas.
- Use more parts of your brain to help remember concepts. Drawing is an excellent way to verify your understanding of complicated concepts, such as cell communication, energy metabolism, or interactions among immune cells. Study the relevant pictures in the text, and try to understand the processes; then, to test yourself, try to draw them out from memory onto a blank piece of paper. Finding the parts of the concept that you cannot remember will be easier because you will get stuck at that particular place in the picture. When studying words, recognizing the parts that you do not know is difficult.
- Try a group review session. Many students find group review sessions to be helpful in checking their thinking and in preparing for examinations. All participants should have already studied the material. Use this group time as a question-and-answer session. Do not rely on notes; try to answer from memory. The Key Questions and Key Points from the text can be used as a guide for formulating quiz questions—or adapt questions from this Study Guide.

Use the Study Guide to Test Yourself

After you have read and studied, answer the pathophysiology questions provided in this study guide. Commit to the answers before you check the key. Testing yourself will help you be a better test taker. Even if you do not think you know the answer to a question, you may be able to figure it out. Sometimes, the only way to find the correct answer is through recognition of the incorrect answers. Score yourself, and review the incorrect answers. Is the answer obvious to you now that you see it? If so, you probably adequately understand the concepts, but you are misreading questions or reading things into the answers. Alternatively, you may not have spent enough time getting the information into your "working knowledge" and still have trouble with retrieval. In this case, more study time is indicated. If you do not understand the question even after seeing the right answer, then you need to go back to the chapter and reread the content until you recognize that the right answer is correct. Your ability to focus on the important material will help improve your test-taking skills with time. Enjoy the challenge!

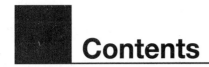

Contents

Introduction to Pathophysiology

TRUE/FALSE

Indicate whether the following statements regarding pathophysiologic concepts are true (T) or false (F).

1. _____ The normal ranges for physiologic parameters such as blood pressure, blood electrolyte levels, and other laboratory tests will vary according to the population studied.

2. _____ Trends and changes in an individual's laboratory values are more reliable than a single observation.

3. _____ There is usually a single, well-defined cause or etiologic factor for a disease process.

4. _____ Pathogenesis refers to the mechanisms whereby an etiologic factor leads to the typically observed clinical manifestations of a disease.

5. _____ Manifestations of a disease process vary among individuals.

6. _____ Epidemiology is the study of patterns of disease among human populations.

7. _____ The principal use of epidemiology is to determine the best way to treat a disease after it occurs in an individual.

8. _____ Most individuals will respond to an identical stressful situation in a similar physiologic manner.

9. _____ Risk factors for a disease are the causes of disease.

10. _____ Health and illness perceptions are affected by individual cultures.

11. _____ A syndrome is a collection of signs and symptoms without a single cause.

12. _____ Clinical manifestations of a disease are constant throughout its clinical course.

13. _____ The prodromal period corresponds to the time during which early signs or symptoms begin to appear.

14. _____ All individuals exposed to a given etiologic factor will develop its associated pathology.

15. _____ Disruption in cellular function and/or communication is the pathophysiologic basis of most diseases.

MULTIPLE CHOICE

Select the one best answer to each of the following questions.

16. Pathophysiology includes all of the following elements *except*
    A. etiology.
    B. clinical manifestations.
    C. mechanisms of pathogenesis.
    D. clinical management.

17. Acquired immunodeficiency syndrome (AIDS) is a disorder in which immune cells are infected with human immunodeficiency virus (HIV) and are subsequently destroyed, leading to increased susceptibility to opportunistic infections. What is the etiologic factor in AIDS?
    A. Increased susceptibility to opportunistic infections
    B. Destruction of immune cells
    C. Human immunodeficiency virus
    D. Acquired immunodeficiency syndrome

1

18. Understanding the epidemiology of a disease is essential for effective
    A. prevention.
    B. therapy.
    C. treatment.
    D. diagnosis.

19. Which of the following is an example of primary prevention?
    A. Childhood immunization for communicable diseases
    B. Routine Papanicolaou (Pap) smear of the cervix
    C. Amniocentesis to detect genetic abnormality in the fetus
    D. Range-of-motion exercises to reverse disuse atrophy in the stroke patient

20. Examples of factors influencing epidemiologic patterns include all of the following *except*
    A. geographic location.
    B. occupation.
    C. socioeconomic status.
    D. political views.

21. Which of the following is an example of a clinical *sign* of disease?
    A. Fatigue
    B. Dizziness
    C. Cough
    D. Pain

22. The development of heart failure from untreated hypertension would be an example of a/an
    A. sequela.
    B. exacerbation.
    C. complication.
    D. chronic phase.

23. Evidence-based treatments are
    A. derived from an understanding of pathophysiology.
    B. based on the results of sound clinical research.
    C. drawn from anecdotal reports about what treatment is effective.
    D. based on personal experience.

FILL IN THE BLANKS

Fill in the blanks with the appropriate word or words.

24. When one is visiting a hospital in another region, differences in laboratory values are likely to be seen because they are based on different _____.

25. The specific cause of some diseases, such as essential hypertension, is unknown, so these conditions are called _____.

26. An undesirable condition that develops because of a treatment is called _____.

27. HIV infection of millions of individuals across several countries is an example of a/an _____.

28. The interval between exposure to a virus and the development of clinical manifestations is called the _____, or _____, period.

29. A/An _____ of rheumatoid arthritis would be associated with an increase in clinical manifestations, whereas the disease is in _____ when these manifestations decrease.

2

30. When the heart rate displayed on a cardiac monitor corresponds to the value obtained when the nurse takes the patient's pulse, the cardiac monitor is said to be a _____ measurement tool.

31. Serum levels of cortisol fluctuate over a 24-hour period, reflecting a _____ _____ rhythm, also known as _____ _____.

32. When a diagnostic test is very good at detecting an abnormality in a patient who actually has the abnormality, it is said to have good _____, whereas a test that does not detect an abnormality in a patient who does not have the abnormality is said to have good _____.

2 Homeostasis, Allostasis, and Adaptive Responses to Stressors

TRUE/FALSE

Indicate whether the following statements regarding homeostasis, allostasis, and stress responses are true (T) or false (F).

1. _____ Homeostasis is a physiologic condition in which systems are functioning at a stable level.

2. _____ Most homeostatic feedback mechanisms function on the principle of negative feedback.

3. _____ Allostasis is a simplified interpretation of homeostasis mechanisms.

4. _____ Many of the signs and symptoms of an acute response to stress are attributable to activation of the sympathetic nervous system.

5. _____ Adaptation to stress is successful when homeostasis is maintained or restored.

6. _____ Selye's three phases of the stress response include alarm, initiation, and resistance.

7. _____ Cortisol is released during the stress response and serves to make more glucose available to the brain.

8. _____ Antidiuretic hormone is released during stress and serves to increase urine output and reduce blood pressure.

9. _____ Hyperplasia of the adrenal cortex, lymphoid atrophy, and stomach ulceration are features of Selye's general adaptation syndrome.

10. _____ The excessive release of cortisol in response to allostatic overload tends to suppress the immune system.

11. _____ Although the central nervous system is known to affect the immune system through various neurotransmitters, the immune system does not affect the central nervous system.

12. _____ All individuals will respond to an identical stressful situation in a similar physiologic manner.

13. _____ Allostatic overload can result in physical and/or psychosocial dysfunction.

14. _____ Epinephrine and norepinephrine are catecholamines released by the sympathetic nervous system and adrenal medulla in response to stress.

15. _____ The goal in caring for patients with stress-related conditions is to eliminate stress.

COMPARE/CONTRAST

16. *The effects of allostatic overload on body organs and systems have been implicated in the pathogenesis of many disorders and disease processes in humans. For each of the physiologic systems below, list three to five disorders that are thought to have a significant stress component.*

Physiologic System	Stress-Induced Disease Process
Nervous system	
Cardiovascular system	
Gastrointestinal system	
Genitourinary system	
Integumentary system	
Respiratory system	
Immune system	
Endocrine system	
Musculoskeletal system	

4

MULTIPLE CHOICE

Select the one best answer to each of the following questions.

17. Which of the following findings would indicate that a patient may be experiencing a "fight-or-flight" reaction to a stressor?
    A. Constricted pupils
    B. Low blood pressure
    C. Increased heart rate
    D. Frequent sighing or yawning

18. In which of Selye's stages of stress response would a patient be if he or she were experiencing gastrointestinal bleeding secondary to peptic ulcer disease?
    A. Alarm
    B. Resistance
    C. Exhaustion
    D. Illness

19. A stressor that stimulates the release of endorphins in the central nervous system is likely to be interpreted as
    A. pleasurable.
    B. painful.
    C. unimportant.
    D. noxious.

20. Several hormones are released during stress and serve to increase blood glucose levels. These include all of the following *except*
    A. cortisol.
    B. growth hormone.
    C. epinephrine.
    D. testosterone.

21. Indicators that a person who is experiencing stress has achieved resistance include
    A. elevated levels of serum cortisol.
    B. heart rate returned to baseline.
    C. sleepiness.
    D. absence of catecholamine secretion.

22. Behavioral indicators that coping is ineffective include all of the following *except*
    A. sleeping more.
    B. major depression.
    C. inability to concentrate.
    D. anorexia.

23. The effects of gender on the stress response are
    A. greatest in the elderly.
    B. related to the effect of sex hormones.
    C. noncontributory.
    D. consistent across the lifespan.

24. Cortisol
    A. is released from the anterior pituitary gland.
    B. has an anabolic effect on somatic muscle.
    C. promotes the creation of glucose from amino acids.
    D. increases lactate formation.

25. Growth hormone release is increased by stress, and one of its effects is
    A. increased glucose availability.
    B. increased protein catabolism.
    C. decreased perception of stress.
    D. decreased endorphin release.

FILL IN THE BLANKS

Fill in the blanks with the appropriate word or words.

26. The three major body systems involved in the stress response are the _____, _____, and _____ systems.

27. A moderate amount of stress is helpful in learning and consolidation of _____.

28. Most of the detrimental effects of chronic stress are attributed to dysregulation of the hormone _____.

29. The biopsychosocial process of change in response to stress is called _____, whereas _____ is usually used for specific behavioral responses to stress.

30. _____ are chemicals released by the brain that cause euphoria, sedation, and elevation of the pain threshold.

31. _____ _____ are an individual's behavioral adaptations to reduce feelings of distress.

32. The release of catecholamines, cortisol, and growth hormone during an acute stress response is helpful because they all increase blood _____ levels to support brain metabolism.

33. Both the _____ and _____ arms of the immune system are suppressed by chronic or prolonged stress.

34. Desensitization involves altering how the _____ responds to selected perceived threats.

UNIT I: Case Studies

Marge is a 42-year-old woman who works full time as a legal secretary and has three children, ages 6, 9, and 11 years. She was divorced 6 months ago and relocated to a new school district. Her children are adjusting to school, but Marge has not established any friendships in the neighborhood. She is in the clinic today with a severe migraine headache that has not responded to her usual ibuprofen medications.

1. According to Selye, because Marge is experiencing severe migraine headaches and is seeking medical care, she is in the stage of
   A. alarm.
   B. resistance.
   C. exhaustion.
   D. symptom emergence.

2. Because stress or allostatic overload is believed to be a significant factor in the etiologic progression of migraine headache, it may be helpful to suggest that Marge
   A. avoid medicating her headaches.
   B. eliminate stressful situations.
   C. cope more effectively.
   D. identify precipitating stressors and initiate preventive measures.

3. Marge indicates that she does not think her migraines are a result of stress because her sister is in a much worse life situation than she is and does not get migraines. Which of the following statements is the best basis for a reply?
   A. Perhaps your sister's situation is not as bad as you think it is.
   B. People respond to stressful situations in different ways.
   C. Migraines are always stress related.
   D. Perhaps your sister has better coping skills.

4. Upon examination, Marge is noted to have elevated blood pressure and heart rate. The most likely explanation for these signs is
   A. excessive release of glucocorticoids.
   B. excessive release of catecholamines.
   C. excessive release of growth hormone.
   D. excessive release of insulin.

Jean is a 28-year-old woman with chronic back pain subsequent to a motor vehicle accident she suffered at age 22. She is currently in the hospital in preparation for back surgery the next day.

5. Jean reports that she seems to have been experiencing colds more frequently since her motor vehicle accident 6 years ago. Considering the physiologic effects of allostatic overload/chronic stress, you know that
   A. the immune system may be suppressed.
   B. this is unrelated to her chronic stress.
   C. excessive secretion of endorphins increases sensitivity to viruses.
   D. the pain medication for her back probably has affected her coping skills.

6. Jean's preoperative laboratory tests show a slightly elevated blood glucose level. This may be attributed to
   A. her normal saline infusion.
   B. increased cortisol release in response to stress.
   C. decreased physical activity while in the hospital.
   D. a side effect of her pain medication.

7. Jean indicates that she would like the television to be turned on to distract her from thinking about the upcoming surgery. This is an example of
   A. ineffective coping.
   B. Selye's stage of exhaustion.
   C. resolving the stressor.
   D. functional coping.

Chapter **2** **Homeostasis, Allostasis, and Adaptive Responses to Stressors**

3 Cell Structure and Function

MATCHING

1. *Match each of the following anatomic terms with the appropriate letter in the figure.*

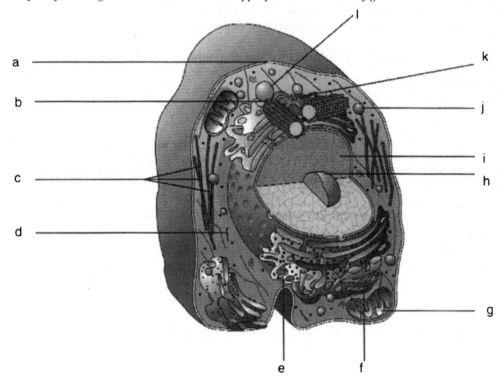

_____ Centrioles

_____ Nucleus

_____ Golgi apparatus

_____ Microtubules

_____ Rough endoplasmic reticulum

_____ Mitochondrion

_____ Plasma membrane

_____ Lysosome

_____ Ribosomes

_____ Secretory granule

_____ Nucleolus

_____ Smooth endoplasmic reticulum

TRUE/FALSE

Indicate whether the following statements regarding cell structure and function are true (T) or false (F).

2. _____ The plasma membrane is composed of a lipid bilayer that is highly permeable to water-soluble and charged molecules.

3. _____ Actin and myosin are proteins that are part of the cellular cytoskeleton.

4. _____ The rough endoplasmic reticulum is the site of synthesis of proteins that are destined for secretion from the cell.

5. _____ Glycolysis occurs within the cell's mitochondria.

6. _____ Large quantities of adenosine triphosphate (ATP) are stored in all cells to provide cellular energy.

7. _____ Glycolysis is an anaerobic process.

8. _____ Oxygen is required to accept low-energy electrons from the mitochondrial electron transport chain enzymes.

9. _____ Channel proteins in the cell membrane allow passive transport of ions.

10. _____ Carrier proteins in the cell membrane are always active transporters.

11. _____ Only cells with voltage-gated ion channels in their plasma membranes are able to conduct action potentials.

12. _____ Movement of large molecules from the extracellular to the intracellular environment is an energy-requiring process.

MULTIPLE CHOICE

Select the one best answer to each of the following questions.

13. The lipids that form the cell membrane are amphipathic (amphiphilic), meaning that they
    A. are insoluble.
    B. have both water-soluble and lipid-soluble parts.
    C. evolved from amphibians.
    D. are synthesized from amino acids.

14. The lipid bilayer can form spontaneously in aqueous solution because
    A. the charge on lipids causes them to attract.
    B. the energy from sunlight is used to move the molecules together.
    C. the lipid bilayer structure allows the water molecules to be less ordered.
    D. the lipid tails form spontaneous covalent bonds.

15. Enzymes function to
    A. increase the speed of chemical reactions.
    B. determine the direction of chemical reactions.
    C. provide the energy to drive chemical reactions.
    D. make energetically unfavorable reactions occur spontaneously.

16. The Gs-protein coupled receptor pathway activates _____ to increase production of cyclic adenosine monophosphate (cAMP).
    A. glycolysis
    B. adenylyl cyclase
    C. phospholipase
    D. phosphodiesterase

Chapter **3 Cell Structure and Function**

17. Cyclic nucleotides, including cAMP and cyclic guanosine monophosphate (cGMP), are degraded by enzymes called
    A. phosphatases.
    B. phosphodiesterases.
    C. lipases.
    D. kinases.

18. Nitric oxide stimulates guanylyl cyclase to produce
    A. diacylglycerol (DAG).
    B. inositol trisphosphate (IP3).
    C. cyclic AMP.
    D. cyclic GMP.

FILL IN THE BLANKS

Fill in the blanks with the appropriate word or words.

19. The energy of the _____ _____ is used by ATP synthase to produce ATP.

20. Cells use _____ receptors to attach to their extracellular matrix.

21. Water always moves passively across cell membranes in response to a/an _____ gradient.

22. The sodium-potassium ion pump transports _____ sodium ions out of the cell in exchange for two potassium ions.

23. The direction of passive ion flux is determined by the _____ gradient.

24. Protein pores that connect the cell cytoplasm of adjacent cells are called _____.

25. Paracrine signaling occurs when signaling molecules travel through the _____ fluid to target cells, whereas endocrine signaling occurs when signaling molecules travel through the _____.

4 Cell Injury, Aging, and Death

Indicate whether the following statements regarding tissue injury are true (T) or false (F).

1. _____ Apoptosis is a cellular process that uses energy to achieve cell death.

2. _____ Apoptosis is always a pathologic process and not a physiologic one.

3. _____ Proteasomes function to degrade intracellular proteins.

4. _____ Metaplasia occurs when a cell type converts to a different cell type in response to chronic injury.

5. _____ The telomere ends of chromosomes get progressively longer with each cell division and contribute to aging.

MULTIPLE CHOICE

Select the one best answer to each of the following questions.

6. Which of the following tissues has a limited capacity for replacement of damaged cells?
   A. Epithelium
   B. Smooth muscle
   C. Connective tissue
   D. Nervous tissue

7. Apoptosis is a physiologic process in which a cell
   A. divides to form two identical daughter cells.
   B. undergoes programmed cell death.
   C. becomes malignant.
   D. converts to a different cell type.

8. Hydropic swelling is a sign of cellular injury associated with
   A. necrosis.
   B. $Na^+ K^+$ pump dysfunction.
   C. apoptosis.
   D. aging.

9. Which of the following is *not* a reversible cellular adaptation?
   A. Atrophy
   B. Hypertrophy
   C. Hyperplasia
   D. Necrosis

10. Glandular tissue normally responds to increased functional demand by
    A. hypertrophy.
    B. hyperplasia.
    C. metaplasia.
    D. neoplasia.

11. Ischemic death of tissue in visceral organs such as the heart typically produces
    A. coagulative necrosis.
    B. liquefactive necrosis.
    C. caseous necrosis.
    D. fat necrosis.

11

12. Cellular injury that results in the production of excessive serum lactate levels is attributable to
    A. immunologic injury.
    B. nutritional injury.
    C. hypoxic injury.
    D. mechanical injury.

13. Age-related changes in body systems can be described as
    A. disease processes.
    B. decreased functional reserve.
    C. reversible injury.
    D. compensatory.

14. When muscle cells decrease in size because of prolonged bed rest, this is called
    A. disuse atrophy.
    B. disuse hypertrophy.
    C. denervation atrophy.
    D. ischemic atrophy.

15. Hypoxia caused by ischemia results in all of the following *except*
    A. reduced ATP production.
    B. lactic acidosis.
    C. hydropic swelling.
    D. increased membrane pump activity.

FILL IN THE BLANKS

Fill in the blanks with the appropriate word or words.

16. _____ _____ and the ability to _____ to changes in the environment are decreased with aging.

17. Insufficient intake of dietary amino acids results in a decreased ability to synthesize _____.

18. Cell injury occurs indirectly when infection activates the _____ _____.

19. Following somatic death, rigor mortis develops because of the accumulation of intracellular _____ in muscle cells.

20. Cell death by _____ often activates the inflammatory response.

5 Genome Structure, Regulation, and Tissue Differentiation

Indicate whether the following statements regarding molecular genetics and cell differentiation are true (T) or false (F).

1. _____ DNA is composed of four nucleotide bases: adenosine, cytosine, uracil, and guanine.

2. _____ Binding of nucleotides is specific such that cytosine (C) always binds with guanine (G).

3. _____ Translation is the process of converting a section of DNA to messenger RNA.

4. _____ Cell division resulting in two daughter cells is known as mitosis.

5. _____ Organization of actin and myosin is identical in all types of muscle cells.

MULTIPLE CHOICE

Select the one best answer to each of the following questions.

6. Cells differ in structure and function because they
   A. all have different DNA and genes.
   B. selectively express certain genes that give them their character.
   C. selectively eliminate certain genes from the genome during development.
   D. undergo selective mutations over time.

7. The critical factor for initiation of gene transcription is
   A. an increase in cellular glucose.
   B. sufficient nutrients.
   C. extracellular signals to initiate the process.
   D. assembly of transcription factors at the promoter area.

8. The endothelium that lines the blood vessels is categorized as
   A. connective tissue.
   B. muscle tissue.
   C. nervous tissue.
   D. epithelial tissue.

9. All of the following nucleotide bases are found in RNA *except*
   A. adenosine.
   B. cytosine.
   C. thymine.
   D. guanosine.

10. A codon is a
    A. section of DNA that is spliced out of the original transcript to form messenger RNA.
    B. sequence of nucleotides found on transfer RNA.
    C. gene.
    D. sequence of three nucleotides that code for an amino acid.

11. The normal human genome consists of
    A. 23 chromosomes.
    B. 22 autosomes and 1 sex chromosome.
    C. 46 chromosomes.
    D. 22 pairs of autosomes.

12. Genes that code for a particular trait come in several forms called
    A. exons.
    B. introns.
    C. alleles.
    D. phenotypes.

13. Examples of connective tissue include
    A. bone marrow.
    B. neuroglia.
    C. skin epithelium.
    D. glands.

14. The processes that allow individual cells to develop into complex organisms include all of the following *except*
    A. cell-to-cell interactions.
    B. cellular mutation.
    C. cellular specialization.
    D. cellular proliferation.

15. Transcription is inhibited by
    A. repressor proteins.
    B. histone proteins.
    C. chromatin proteins.
    D. ribosomal proteins.

FILL IN THE BLANKS

Fill in the blanks with the appropriate word or words.

16. It is estimated that the human genome contains approximately _____ genes.

17. Strands of deoxyribonucleotides are linked into polymers by bonds between _____.

18. Synthesis of mRNA from the DNA template is termed _____.

19. Cells capable of cell division (mitosis) are called _____ cells.

20. The four major tissue types are _____, _____, _____, and _____.

21. If a sequence of DNA is formed by the nucleotides CATGGTACGGAATT, then the complementary sequence of DNA would be _____, and the complementary sequence of RNA would be _____.

22. Replication of DNA is accomplished by the enzyme _____ _____, whereas transcription of DNA is accomplished by the enzyme _____ _____.

23. The 64 different codons code for _____ different amino acids.

24. Traits that are transmitted to offspring but are not coded by inherited gene sequences are called _____.

25. The amino acids that form proteins can be assigned to three different categories based on their chemical solubility properties: _____, _____, and _____.

Chapter **5** **Genome Structure, Regulation, and Tissue Differentiation**

6 Genetic and Developmental Disorders

Indicate whether the following statements regarding genetic disorders are true (T) or false (F).

1. _____ Genetic diseases resulting from mitochondrial gene mutations are transmitted from mother to offspring.

2. _____ The paternal source of an abnormal gene (mother or father) makes no difference to the effect of a mutation on the offspring.

3. _____ Congenital disorders are always genetic disorders.

4. _____ Gene therapy is available for most genetic disorders.

5. _____ Multifactorial genetic disorders are more common in the population than are single-gene disorders.

MULTIPLE CHOICE

Select the one best answer to each of the following questions.

6. A mutation caused by the substitution of one DNA nucleotide for another is called a
   A. point mutation.
   B. frameshift mutation.
   C. codon mutation.
   D. single-gene mutation.

7. Genetic disorders that follow predictable patterns of inheritance are called
   A. polygenic disorders.
   B. chromosomal aneuploidy.
   C. nonmendelian disorders.
   D. single-gene disorders.

8. Which of the following chromosomal disorders is categorized as a monosomy?
   A. Klinefelter syndrome
   B. Down syndrome
   C. Turner syndrome
   D. Cri du chat syndrome

9. Characteristics of autosomal-dominant disorders include the fact that
   A. offspring of an affected individual have a 25% chance of being carriers.
   B. offspring of an affected individual have a 25% chance of inheriting the disease.
   C. males are affected more often than females.
   D. unaffected individuals do not transmit the disease.

10. Individuals affected with which genetic disorder are almost always males?
    A. Autosomal-dominant disorders
    B. Autosomal-recessive disorders
    C. Chromosomal disorders
    D. X-linked disorders

11. The acronym TORCH refers to infectious diseases that may be teratogenic and include all of the following *except*
    A. toxoplasmosis.
    B. rubella.
    C. chickenpox.
    D. herpes.

12. The fetus is most vulnerable to teratogenic influences during
    A. delivery.
    B. conception.
    C. gestational weeks 1 to 3.
    D. gestational weeks 3 to 9.

13. Which of the following would be a significant risk factor for having a fetus with Down syndrome?
    A. Family history of autosomal genetic disorders
    B. Advanced maternal age (>35 years)
    C. Exposure to rubella in the second trimester
    D. Perinatal hypoxemia

MATCHING

Match the following genetic abnormalities with their mode of inheritance. Answers may be used more than once.

14. _____ Turner syndrome

15. _____ Klinefelter syndrome

16. _____ Huntington chorea

17. _____ Marfan disease

18. _____ Hemophilia A and B

19. _____ Phenylketonuria

20. _____ Down syndrome

21. _____ Cystic fibrosis

22. _____ Hypertension

A. Autosomal-dominant
B. Autosomal-recessive
C. X-linked
D. Chromosomal aneuploidy
E. Multifactorial

FILL IN THE BLANKS

Fill in the blanks with the appropriate word or words.

23. When duplicated homologous chromosomes pair up and exchange sections of DNA during meiosis, this is called

    _____.

24. When duplicated chromosomes fail to separate during meiosis, this is called _____.

25. The _____ arm of a chromosome is called p, and the _____ arm is called q.

26. The probability of a father transmitting an X-linked disorder, such as hemophilia, to his son is _____.

7 Neoplasia

Indicate whether the following statements regarding neoplastic disorders are true (T) or false (F).

1. _____ In general, a grade I tumor histology determination has a worse prognosis than a grade IV determination.

2. _____ The underlying cause of cancer is genetic mutations in growth control genes.

3. _____ Factors that are mutagenic are likely to be carcinogenic.

4. _____ Excess activity of the *Rb* retinoblastoma gene increases the risk of developing cancer.

5. _____ With appropriate lifestyle choices, it is possible to eliminate exposure to carcinogens.

6. _____ Proto-oncogenes code for growth factors, growth receptors, and intracellular growth pathway components.

7. _____ Some tumor suppression genes code for DNA repair enzymes.

8. _____ Lung cancer is the most prevalent form of cancer in the United States

9. _____ Lung cancer is the deadliest form of cancer in the United States.

10. _____ Any evidence of local invasiveness of a tumor means it is malignant.

11. _____ Carcinoma in situ is a benign form of tumor growth.

12. _____ Metastasis is nearly always a fatal outcome of cancer.

MULTIPLE CHOICE

Select the one best answer to each of the following questions.

13. Proto-oncogene overexpression is associated with the development of
    A. birth defects.
    B. X-linked genetic defects.
    C. congenital disease.
    D. cancer.

14. The most important differentiating feature between benign and malignant tumors is
    A. invasiveness.
    B. a difference in the rate of cell growth within the tumor.
    C. a difference in the tissue of origin.
    D. the size of the tumor.

15. Which of the following tumors is malignant?
    A. Adenoma
    B. Fibroma
    C. Carcinoma
    D. Osteoma

16. Cancer cells exhibit all of the following properties *except*
    A. immortality.
    B. excessive proliferation.
    C. nomadic.
    D. high differentiation.

17. Proto-oncogene overactivity may increase cellular proliferation through all of the following mechanisms *except*
    A. excessive production of growth factors.
    B. excessive production of growth factor receptors.
    C. excessive production of transcription factors.
    D. excessive production of p53.

18. Tumor suppression genes contribute to cancer when they are
    A. overproduced in the cell.
    B. overactive in the cell.
    C. absent from the cell.
    D. present in more than one location on the chromosome.

19. Full expression of cancer in a host is a multistep phenomenon. These steps include all of the following *except*
    A. initiation.
    B. promotion.
    C. progression.
    D. emigration.

20. Telomerase is an enzyme that
    A. allows cancer cells to metastasize.
    B. is essential for normal cellular function.
    C. contributes to immortality of cancer cells.
    D. initiates apoptosis.

21. Tumor "grade" refers to which property of the cancer cells?
    A. Location in the body
    B. Degree of local invasiveness
    C. Extent of metastasis
    D. Histologic characteristics

22. Tumor staging is a process whereby
    A. the location of tumors in the body is determined.
    B. all of the tumors are removed from the body.
    C. tumor cell characteristics are analyzed under the microscope.
    D. the tissue of origin is biochemically determined.

23. If a tumor is characterized according to the tumor, node, metastasis (TNM) system as T2 N1 M0, what is the correct interpretation?
    A. Tumor is localized with no lymph node involvement or metastasis.
    B. Tumor is locally invasive with regional lymph node involvement; there is no metastasis.
    C. Tumor has spread to distant lymph nodes; there is no metastasis.
    D. Tumor is disseminated to lymph nodes and distant sites.

24. What type of tissue cells are the source of cancer cells?
    A. Morphogenic cells
    B. Stem cells
    C. Terminally differentiated cells
    D. Embryonic cells

25. *Compare and contrast the features of benign and malignant tumors by filling in the table below.*

Characteristic	Benign Tumors	Malignant Tumors
Conventional terminology		
Histology		
Proliferation rate		
Metastasis		
Necrosis within the tumor		
Recurrence after treatment		
Prognosis		

UNIT II: Case Studies

Mr. and Mrs. Frank are planning to conceive a child and are interested in receiving genetic counseling because of their ages and a history of cystic fibrosis on Mrs. Frank's side of the family. A brief history reveals that Mr. Frank has no known family history of cystic fibrosis or any other genetic disorder. He is 45 years old and has two children from a previous marriage, both of whom are well. Mrs. Frank has a sister with three children the last of whom was diagnosed with cystic fibrosis. There are no other known family members with this disease. Mrs. Frank is 35 years old and has no children.

1. When assessing the risk for bearing a child with cystic fibrosis, one must consider that the disease is genetically inherited as
   A. autosomal-dominant.
   B. autosomal-recessive.
   C. X-linked.
   D. chromosomal.

2. Assuming the worst-case scenario, which is that both Mr. and Mrs. Frank have the defective gene for cystic fibrosis, what is the probability of their bearing an affected child?
   A. No risk
   B. 50%
   C. 25%
   D. 75%

3. Mr. and Mrs. Frank decide to undergo genetic testing to determine whether either of them has the cystic fibrosis gene. Mr. Frank does not have it, but Mrs. Frank is heterozygous for the gene (one normal gene, one cystic fibrosis gene). With this knowledge, one can assess the risk of their bearing a child affected by cystic fibrosis to be closest to
   A. near 0%.
   B. 50%.
   C. 25%.
   D. 75%.

4. Because of their ages, Mr. and Mrs. Frank are concerned about bearing a child with Down syndrome (trisomy 21) and would like genetic testing to determine their risk prior to initiating the pregnancy. Can this be done?
   A. No, Down syndrome can only be detected after conception.
   B. Yes, Down syndrome risk can be detected by parental blood analysis.

5. After Mrs. Frank becomes pregnant, she undergoes amniocentesis to analyze the fetal karyotype. The results indicate that the fetus has two 21st chromosomes. What is the most accurate interpretation of this result?
   A. The child is normal.
   B. Down syndrome is unlikely.
   C. There are no genetic abnormalities.
   D. There are no congenital abnormalities.

Sam is a 72-year-old man who is in the clinic with complaints of urinary retention, difficulty initiating the urinary stream, and dribbling. These symptoms are believed by the examining clinician to be associated with an enlarged prostate.

6. A blood sample for prostate-specific antigen (PSA) is obtained. PSA is a
   A. tumor marker for prostate cancer.
   B. histologic examination of the prostate cells.
   C. test for the presence of metastasis.
   D. test for prostate infection (prostatitis).

7. The PSA value is abnormally elevated, and Sam is scheduled for a prostate biopsy procedure. The purpose of the biopsy is to
   A. obtain tumor cells for histologic examination and grading.
   B. determine whether the tumor cells have invaded locally or metastasized.
   C. stage the tumor.
   D. determine how much of the prostate is cancerous.

8. The results of the biopsy indicate that Sam has "anaplastic cells." This means that
   A. the tumor cells are benign.
   B. the tumor cells are malignant.
   C. the tumor has already spread to distant sites.
   D. the tumor is well differentiated.

9. Next, Sam is scheduled for a staging procedure to determine the extent of disease. The oncologist notes in the chart that Sam's stage is T1 N0 M0, indicating that
   A. the tumor has spread beyond the prostate.
   B. there is only regional metastasis.
   C. the tumor is localized within the prostate gland.
   D. the tumor is local and benign.

10. Based on the grading and staging procedures, it is determined that Sam should be treated with surgery to relieve the problem of urinary obstruction, followed by localized irradiation of the prostate gland. Irradiation of the prostate will
    A. selectively kill the tumor cells.
    B. enhance the ability of immune cells to detect and destroy tumor cells.
    C. kill all cells in the irradiated region.
    D. kill the most rapidly dividing cells in the irradiated region.

Sandy is a 36-year-old woman with a strong family history of breast cancer, affecting her mother, sister, and three maternal aunts before the age of 50. Sandy's sister was just diagnosed at age 38, and Sandy is concerned that she may have a genetic predisposition to the disease. A clinical breast examination reveals no significant lumps; however, the breasts are dense and difficult to examine. Sandy is scheduled for a mammography and for genetic testing for BRCAI and BRCAII.

11. The *BRCAI* and *BRCAII* genes are associated with an inherited form of breast cancer accounting for about 5% of breast cancers. These genes are classified as
    A. proto-oncogenes.
    B. oncogenes.
    C. tumor suppression genes.
    D. malignancy genes.

12. Sandy's genetic test results indicate that she does not have an abnormality of the *BRCAI* or *BRCAII* gene, but her mammogram reveals a suspicious lesion in the upper outer quadrant of the left breast. Which of the following statements should guide further testing?
    A. Breast cancer is unlikely in view of *BRCA* gene results.
    B. Breast cancer is inevitable in view of the family history.
    C. Breast cancer is possible, and evaluation of the breast mass is required.
    D. Breast cancer is possible, and further genetic testing is advised.

13. Sandy is very upset about the mammography findings and wants further testing to be done immediately. She undergoes a biopsy procedure, the result of which reveals anaplasia of the sample cells. This means
A. metastatic breast cancer is present.
B. benign fibrocystic cells are present.
C. the breast lesion contains malignant cells.
D. tumor cells have invaded locally.

14. Sandy is scheduled for surgery to remove the breast lump and evaluate the regional lymph nodes. Her cancer is categorized according to the TNM system as T2 N2 M0 (stage IIIA). This means that
A. tumor in situ is present.
B. several regional lymph nodes are involved.
C. extensive metastasis is present.
D. bilateral breast disease is present.

15. After surgery, Sandy is scheduled to receive several rounds of chemotherapy. Chemotherapy is usually administered in cycles because
A. cancer cells are in different phases of the cell cycle.
B. it takes several courses to reach an adequate blood level.
C. larger doses can be used during each cycle.
D. cancer cells become more sensitive to the drugs over time.

8 | Infectious Processes

MATCHING

Match the microorganism on the left with its descriptor on the right. Answers may be used more than once or not at all.

1. _____ *Streptococcus pneumoniae*	A. Retrovirus
2. _____ Histoplasmosis	B. DNA virus
	C. Fungus
3. _____ Human immunodeficiency virus	D. Gram-negative bacterial rod
4. _____ Scabies	E. Bacterial coccus
	F. Anaerobe
5. _____ Helminths (worms)	G. Parasite
6. _____ Tinea	
7. _____ Epstein-Barr virus	
8. _____ *Escherichia coli*	
9. _____ *Clostridium botulinum*	
10. _____ *Candida*	

MULTIPLE CHOICE

Select the one best answer to each of the following questions.

11. Opportunistic infections occur when
    A. virulent pathogens infect the host.
    B. resident flora cause infectious disease.
    C. bacteria are spread by poor handwashing.
    D. transient bacteria spread among hospitalized patients.

12. The chain of infection between the organism's reservoir and the victim can be broken at any of the following points *except*
    A. the portal of entry.
    B. the portal of exit.
    C. immunization.
    D. the mode of transmission.

13. Microbial virulence refers to the microbe's ability to
    A. gain access to a host.
    B. cause illness.
    C. prevent opsonization.
    D. secrete endotoxins.

14. The Gram stain reaction
    A. illuminates cell walls of parasites.
    B. is used with fungi.
    C. identifies RNA and DNA viruses.
    D. differentiates between two groups of bacteria.

22

15. A large number of organisms inhabit humans on an ongoing manner, generally not causing disease. These are called
    A. commensal.
    B. opportunist.
    C. codependent.
    D. habitant.

16. The development of resistance to antibiotics frequently occurs because of
    A. excessive exposure of organisms to antibiotics.
    B. random genetic mutations that alter microbial resistance characteristics.
    C. the ability of microorganisms to purposefully alter their genes.
    D. the direct transfer of genetic resistance from one organism to another.

17. The most effective method to limit the transmission of infection is
    A. handwashing.
    B. using tissues if coughing.
    C. administering prophylactic antibiotics.
    D. encouraging patients to eat.

FILL IN THE BLANKS

Fill in the blanks with the appropriate word or words.

18. Epidemiology is the study of the distribution of disease in a defined _____.

19. The transmission of an infection from one person to another requires five unbroken events in a chain. These are:

    _____, _____, _____, _____, and _____.

20. An inanimate object such as a contaminated eating utensil that participates in the transmission of infection is called

    a _____.

21. Certain characteristics increase the risk for contracting an infection and should prompt diligence in prevention and

    assessment for infection. These include _____ and _____.

22. When no signs or symptoms of disease are present, the presence of microorganisms on the skin and mucous mem-

    branes is called _____.

23. The microorganisms that affect humans can be grouped into four broad categories:_____, _____,

    _____, and _____.

24. Most microorganisms that infect humans remain in the extracellular space; however, _____ must gain
    entry into cells to establish an infection.

25. The microorganisms that inhabit the gastrointestinal tract may alter the host's _____.

9 Inflammation and Immunity

LABELING

1. On the diagram below, indicate the blood cell types that evolve from the myeloid and the lymphoid lineages. Include B cells, T cells, red blood cells, platelets, monocytes, and granulocytes (neutrophils, eosinophils, and basophils).

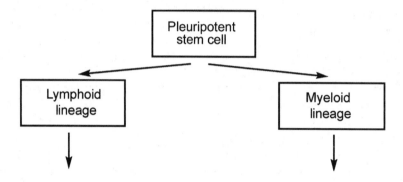

2. On the antibody shown below, indicate the Fab and Fc portions. Label the light and heavy chains. Indicate where the antibody binds its antigen.

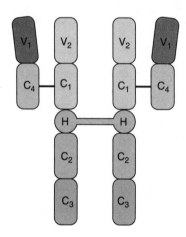

Indicate whether the following statements regarding the anatomy and physiology of the immune system are true (T) or false (F).

3. _____ The primary lymphoid organs are the bone marrow and thymus.

4. _____ The lymphocyte is the most numerous white blood cell (WBC) type in the peripheral blood.

5. _____ The number of neutrophils in the blood increases during acute bacterial infection.

6. _____ Macrophages are mature monocytes.

7. _____ Mast cells are closely related in structure and function to basophils.

8. _____ An increase in neutrophil bands is commonly used as an indicator of acute bacterial infection.

9. _____ T lymphocytes are the principal agents of humoral immunity.

10. _____ Lymphocytes that have CD4 receptors on their cell surface are called T helper cells.

11. _____ B lymphocytes are the principal agents of antibody-mediated immunity.

12. _____ Cytokines are intercellular communication peptides secreted by cells.

13. _____ Previous exposure to foreign antigens is required for activation of neutrophils.

14. _____ Neutrophils marginate along the capillary wall by binding to chemokines and selectin receptors.

15. _____ Interleukin-1 (IL-1), IL-6, and tumor necrosis factor-a (TNF-a) are mediators of inflammation.

16. _____ Cytotoxic T cells bind antigen displayed on cellular major histocompatibility complex (MHC) class II proteins.

17. _____ B cells function as antigen-presenting cells, displaying antigen on their MHC II proteins.

MULTIPLE CHOICE

Select the one best answer to each of the following questions.

18. All of the following structures are considered secondary lymphoid organs *except*
   A. the spleen.
   B. the tonsils.
   C. the bone marrow.
   D. the lymph glands.

19. When used in reference to the WBC differential, a "shift to the left" means
   A. an increase in total WBC count.
   B. an increase in segmented neutrophils.
   C. an increase in neutrophil bands.
   D. an increase in immature lymphocyte blast cells.

20. A normal total WBC count ranges from about
   A. 4000 to 10,000 cells/μL.
   B. 1500 to 3000 cells/μL.
   C. 10,000 to 15,000 cells/μL.
   D. 500 to 1000 cells/μL.

21. The normal percentage of neutrophils in the WBC count is about
   A. 20%.
   B. 40%.
   C. 70%.
   D. 90%.

22. The WBCs that migrate to a site of infection quickly are
    A. monocytes.
    B. lymphocytes.
    C. macrophages.
    D. neutrophils.

23. Basophils and mast cells are unique in that they
    A. bind and display IgE antibodies on their surfaces.
    B. secrete cytokines.
    C. are nonspecific.
    D. release mediators that enhance inflammation.

24. Macrophages have several roles in the inflammatory and immune response, which include all of the following functions *except*
    A. phagocytosis and antigen presentation.
    B. synthesis of serum antibodies.
    C. secretion of inflammatory cytokines.
    D. sentry functions for detection of foreign antigens.

25. Activation of the complement cascade by the classic pathway begins with
    A. interaction of C3 and foreign antigen.
    B. C1 binding to the antigen–antibody complex.
    C. aggregation of C6789 to form the membrane attack complex.
    D. interaction of C1 with foreign antibody.

26. Classic local manifestations of inflammation include all of the following *except*
    A. coolness.
    B. redness.
    C. swelling.
    D. pain.

27. When inflammation is chronic, the predominant cell type is
    A. basophil.
    B. lymphocyte.
    C. neutrophil.
    D. granulocyte.

28. The type of inflammatory exudate characterized as thick, sticky, and high in protein is termed
    A. serous exudate.
    B. fibrinous exudate.
    C. purulent exudate.
    D. hemorrhagic exudate.

29. Which of the following findings is a systemic sign of inflammation?
    A. Pain
    B. Loss of function
    C. Elevated C-reactive protein
    D. Swelling

30. The malaise, fever, and increase in acute-phase proteins that occur with inflammation are attributed to increases in
    A. activated complement.
    B. IL-1, IL-6, and TNF-α.
    C. bacterial toxins.
    D. neutrophils.

Chapter **9** Inflammation and Immunity

Copyright © 2019, Elsevier Inc. All rights reserved.

31. Specific immunity refers to functions of
    A. natural killer cells.
    B. the mononuclear phagocyte system.
    C. mast cells.
    D. B lymphocytes and T lymphocytes.

32. Antigens displayed in association with major histocompatibility complex (MHC) I complexes on the cell surface are usually
    A. bacterial in origin.
    B. obtained from intracellular proteins.
    C. obtained by phagocytosis.
    D. bound to antibodies.

33. Lymphocytes that have CD8 proteins on their cell surface are categorized as
    A. cytotoxic.
    B. helper.
    C. natural killer.
    D. B cells.

34. T helper cells can recognize an antigen when
    A. it is displayed on the cell surface in association with MHC I.
    B. it circulates in the blood or lymph.
    C. it is displayed on the cell surface in association with MHC II.
    D. it is bound to antibody.

35. Plasma cells secrete
    A. inflammatory cytokines.
    B. complement.
    C. TNF-α.
    D. antibodies.

36. Antibody class is determined by
    A. the structure of the Fab region.
    B. the structure of the Fc region.
    C. the structure of the B-cell receptor.
    D. the structure of the light chain.

37. The first type of antibody to be secreted on initial exposure to an antigen is
    A. IgA.
    B. IgG.
    C. IgE.
    D. IgM.

38. All of the following antibodies are monomers *except*
    A. IgD.
    B. IgG.
    C. IgE.
    D. IgM.

39. Plasma cells are
    A. specialized natural killer cells.
    B. antibody-secreting B lymphocytes.
    C. activated monocytes.
    D. precursors of platelets.

40. Which is an example of passive immunity?
    A. Response to vaccination
    B. Response to disease
    C. Placental transfer of antibodies
    D. Transplant rejection

41. Which of the following immune responses requires T helper cell assistance?
    A. B-cell clonal proliferation
    B. Activation of the complement cascade
    C. Effective phagocytosis by neutrophils
    D. Macrophage chemotaxis and phagocytosis

42. The antigen-binding specificity of B cells and T cells is determined
    A. in response to foreign antigen.
    B. randomly, by genetic recombination during development.
    C. by unknown mechanisms.
    D. by antigen-presenting cells.

43. Which of the following situations represents a breach in the "first line of defense" against infection?
    A. An abnormally low total WBC count
    B. A "shift to the right" on the WBC differential
    C. Use of an indwelling bladder catheter
    D. Poor nutritional status

FILL IN THE BLANKS

Fill in the blanks with the appropriate word or words.

44. Macrophages display numerous receptors on their cell surfaces that help them localize antigens. Some of these receptors bind to opsins, such as the _____ and _____ receptors, whereas others bind directly to microorganisms, including the _____ and _____ receptors.

45. The subtype of helper T cell called TH_2 releases a cytokine called interleukin-4, which stimulates B cells to produce the _____ type of antibody.

46. Label the following steps of antigen presentation.

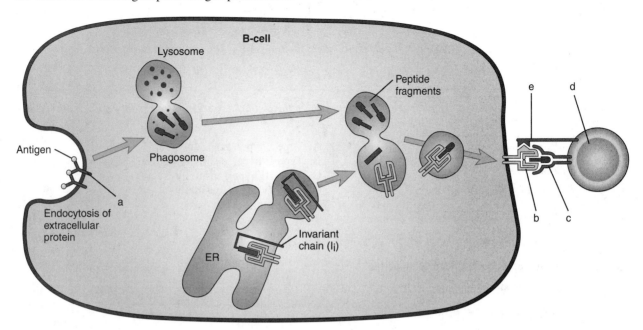

_____ Helper T cell

_____ MHC II protein

_____ B-cell receptor

_____ CD4 protein

_____ T-cell receptor

10 Alterations in Immune Function

MATCHING

Match the disorder on the left with its pathogenetic mechanism on the right. Answers may be used more than once. Some disorders have two answers.

1. _____ Rheumatoid arthritis
2. _____ Asthma
3. _____ Graves disease
4. _____ Hemolytic disease of the newborn
5. _____ Contact dermatitis
6. _____ Poststreptococcal glomerulonephritis
7. _____ Type 1 diabetes mellitus
8. _____ Systemic lupus erythematosus
9. _____ Allergic rhinitis
10. _____ Myasthenia gravis

A. Type I hypersensitivity
B. Type II hypersensitivity
C. Type III hypersensitivity
D. Type IV hypersensitivity
E. Autoimmune

MULTIPLE CHOICE

Select the one best answer to each of the following questions.

11. Certain genotypes have been shown to be associated with a higher risk of developing autoimmune diseases. These genes are of the class
    A. major histocompatibility complex (MHC) genes.
    B. T-cell receptor genes.
    C. B-cell antibody genes.
    D. interleukin (IL) genes.

12. Antibodies are the mediators of all of the hypersensitivity reactions *except*
    A. the type I (anaphylactic) reaction.
    B. the type II (cytotoxic) reaction.
    C. the type III (immune complex) reaction.
    D. the type IV (delayed) reaction.

13. The antibody type IgE is involved in which type of hypersensitivity reaction?
    A. Type I (anaphylactic) reaction
    B. Type II (cytotoxic) reaction
    C. Type III (immune complex) reaction
    D. Type IV (delayed) reaction

14. Graft-versus-host disease is an example of a
    A. type I (anaphylactic) reaction.
    B. type II (cytotoxic) reaction.
    C. type III (immune complex) reaction.
    D. type IV (delayed) reaction.

15. Severe combined immunodeficiency is a disorder of
    A. T-cell dysfunction resulting from thymus agenesis.
    B. selective B-cell abnormality.
    C. lymphocyte stem cell failure.
    D. absent white blood cell growth factors.

16. Chronic stress may cause secondary immunosuppression due to
    A. overstimulation of the bone marrow, leading to failure.
    B. overproduction of cortisol.
    C. impaired antibody production.
    D. excessive catecholamine release.

17. Alterations in immune function may be related to nutritional deficits or excesses. An example of this is
    A. deficiencies in vitamin B_{12} affect production of antibodies.
    B. excessive fat intake decreases overall lymphocyte production.
    C. insufficient calorie and protein intake results in decreased numbers and function of T cells.
    D. adequate amounts of zinc and folate are required for granulocyte maturation.

18. Aging affects the immune system in all of the following ways *except*
    A. reduced T-cell function.
    B. hyper-reactivity to new antigens.
    C. decrease in antibody production.
    D. diminished T-cell proliferation.

19. Severe combined immunodeficiency disorders
    A. are usually caused by autosomal-recessive anomalies.
    B. only affect T-cell functioning.
    C. rarely present prior to 12 to 18 months of age.
    D. are transitory and require no interventions.

FILL IN THE BLANKS

Fill in the blanks with the appropriate word or words.

20. Most autoimmune disorders are mediated through type _____ or _____ hypersensitivity mechanisms.

21. Environmental triggers for autoimmune diseases include _____ and occupational or environmental _____.

22. _____ is a therapy for some autoimmune diseases where _____ are removed and replaced with colloid solutions.

23. Hemolytic disease of the newborn (erythroblastosis fetalis) is an example of a type _____ hypersensitivity reaction between the mother's Rh-positive _____ and subsequent fetal Rh-positive red blood cells.

24. Immunodeficiency disorders can be categorized as primary or secondary. Categorize each of the following disorders as primary (P) or secondary (S).

    _____ HIV/AIDS

    _____ Malnutrition

    _____ Chemotherapy

    _____ Severe combined immunodeficiency

    _____ DiGeorge syndrome

    _____ Selective IgA deficiency

11 Malignant Disorders of White Blood Cells

TRUE/FALSE

Indicate whether the following statements regarding malignant disorders of white blood cells (WBCs) are true (T) or false (F).

1. _____ The Philadelphia chromosome results from a balanced translocation that forms a new gene called *bcr-abl*.

2. _____ The term *clinical remission* is synonymous with *cure*.

3. _____ Plasma cell myeloma is characterized by high serum levels of a monoclonal antibody.

4. _____ In general, the non-Hodgkin lymphomas have a better prognosis for cure than does Hodgkin disease.

5. _____ The most important determinant of prognosis for lymphoma is the histologic grade of the tumor.

MULTIPLE CHOICE

Select the one best answer to each of the following questions.

6. Leukemia is characterized by
   A. overproduction of blasts in the bone marrow.
   B. overproduction of malignant plasma cells.
   C. the presence of Reed-Sternberg cells.
   D. overproduction of monoclonal antibodies.

7. Generally speaking, the type of leukemia with the best prognosis for cure is
   A. acute lymphocytic leukemia.
   B. acute myelogenous leukemia.
   C. chronic lymphocytic leukemia.
   D. chronic myelogenous leukemia.

8. The most common cause of death in patients with leukemic disease is
   A. hemorrhage.
   B. infection.
   C. neurotoxicity from chemotherapeutic agents.
   D. cardiac failure.

9. Manifestations of *untreated* acute leukemia include all of the following *except*
   A. a low total WBC count.
   B. a low platelet count.
   C. anemia.
   D. bone pain.

10. An important diagnostic feature of chronic myelogenous leukemia is the presence of
    A. more than 30% blast cells in the peripheral blood.
    B. total WBC counts exceeding 75,000 cells/mL.
    C. the Philadelphia chromosome.
    D. infiltration of bony structures.

11. Non-Hodgkin lymphoma is characterized by
    A. a contiguous, predictable pattern of spreading.
    B. the presence of Reed-Sternberg cells on histologic examination.
    C. painless lymph node enlargement.
    D. rare metastasis.

32

12. Hodgkin disease most commonly presents with
    A. an enlarged, painless cervical lymph node.
    B. an enlarged, painful lymph node.
    C. an elevated total WBC count.
    D. an increase in Reed-Sternberg cells in the peripheral blood.

13. Bence Jones proteins are indicators of
    A. leukemia.
    B. Hodgkin disease.
    C. non-Hodgkin lymphoma.
    D. plasma cell myeloma.

14. For which of the following diseases is radiation therapy most appropriate?
    A. Acute leukemia
    B. Chronic leukemia
    C. Hodgkin disease
    D. Multiple myeloma

15. Non-Hodgkin lymphoma includes cells of all the following types *except*
    A. natural killer cells.
    B. granulocytes.
    C. T cells.
    D. B cells.

FILL IN THE BLANKS

Fill in the blanks with the appropriate word or words.

16. In some cases, a malignant lymphoid cell type presents as lymphoma, whereas in other cases, it presents as leukemia.

    The difference between lymphoma and leukemia is considered to be a difference in _____ of the disease.

17. Categorize each of the following hematologic cell malignancies either myeloid (M) or lymphoid (L):

    _____ Acute monocytic leukemia

    _____ Acute promyelocytic leukemia

    _____ Burkitt lymphoma

    _____ Chronic neutrophilic leukemia

    _____ Polycythemia vera

    _____ Plasma cell myeloma

    _____ Hodgkin disease

18. Few chemicals have been found to be definitely associated with leukemia; these include _____, _____, _____, and _____ found in certain foods.

19. The bone marrow suppression associated with hematologic malignancies commonly produces _____, _____, and _____.

20. Bone marrow transplantation may use a patient's own stem cells, called _____ transplant, or those of a closely related family member, called _____ transplant.

12 HIV Disease and AIDS

MATCHING

1. Match each of the following terms with the appropriate letter in the figure:

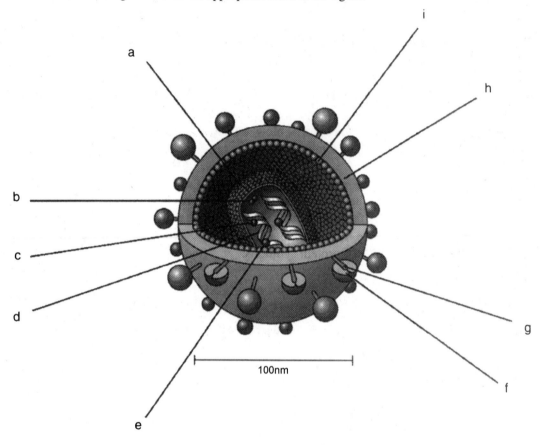

100nm

_____ p24 capsid   _____ Integrase

_____ Reverse transcriptase   _____ gp41

_____ p17 matrix   _____ Protease

_____ RNA   _____ gp120

_____ Lipid bilayer

TRUE/FALSE

Indicate whether the following statements regarding human immunodeficiency virus (HIV) and acquired immunodeficiency syndrome (AIDS) are true (T) or false (F).

2. _____ Heterosexual contact with infected partners is the most common route of HIV transmission in Africa and Southeast Asia.

3. _____ With appropriate highly active antiretroviral therapy, HIV can be eradicated from the body and cure is likely.

4. _____ Condoms and abstinence are the only contraceptive methods that are effective in preventing transmission of HIV.

5. _____ A high maternal viral load of HIV increases the risk of transmission to the fetus.

6. _____ An effective vaccine is available to prevent HIV infection in humans.

MULTIPLE CHOICE

Select the one best answer to each of the following questions.

7. Which of the following exposures represents the greatest risk for acquiring HIV?
   A. A blood splash from an HIV-infected individual onto intact skin
   B. Perinatal transmission from an HIV-infected mother to her fetus
   C. Receiving a blood transfusion from a U.S. blood bank
   D. Heterosexual contact using latex condoms

8. HIV virus is called a retrovirus because it
   A. contains DNA that must be synthesized into RNA to form new virus.
   B. enters the cell in a reverse fashion through the CD4 receptor.
   C. contains the enzyme reverse transcriptase.
   D. reverses the usual sequence of protein synthesis.

9. HIV primarily infects T helper cells and macrophages because
   A. they have CD4 receptors on their cell surfaces.
   B. other cells do not have the internal machinery to produce a new virus.
   C. they are phagocytic and engulf the virus.
   D. the virus knows that these cells must be destroyed to ensure its survival.

10. Some people are resistant to HIV infection because
    A. they do not have CD4 receptors on their T helper cells.
    B. they lack one or more necessary coreceptors for viral binding and insertion.
    C. their immune systems are stronger.
    D. they were exposed to HIV-like viruses and have developed immunity.

11. Which of the following HIV-positive individuals would appropriately be given the diagnosis of AIDS?
    A. One who developed oral candidiasis
    B. One with a CD4 count of 250 cells/μL
    C. One with *Pneumocystis jiroveci* pneumonia
    D. One with a herpetic outbreak on the genitalia

12. The HIV virus is known to mutate frequently within an infected individual. This is because
    A. the virus is trying to escape immune detection.
    B. reverse transcriptase has poor fidelity and makes errors in transcription.
    C. the rate of viral production is so fast that errors in assembly occur.
    D. the selective pressure of antiretroviral drugs increases the mutation rate.

13. Protease inhibitors work by
    A. blocking the protein binding between glycoprotein (gp) 120 and CD4.
    B. inhibiting reverse transcriptase activity.
    C. inhibiting translation of viral mRNA into protein.
    D. inhibiting protein splicing, viral assembly, and maturation.

14. The vast majority of HIV/AIDS cases in the world today are found in
    A. the United States.
    B. sub-Saharan Africa.
    C. Europe.
    D. Asia.

15. Long-term survival of individuals with HIV infection is associated with all of the following *except*
    A. inheriting a mutant *CCR5* gene.
    B. high CD4 cell count.
    C. increased antibody production.
    D. low viral load.

FILL IN THE BLANKS

Fill in the blanks with the appropriate word or words.

16. More than one genotype of HIV virus has been identified; however, the great majority of HIV-infected individuals in the United States, Europe, Australia, and Central Africa have HIV type _____.

17. Several categories of drugs are used to inhibit the HIV lifecycle. These are

    1. _____

    2. _____

    3. _____

    4. _____

    5. _____

18. An HIV-positive individual is diagnosed with AIDS if the CD4+ lymphocyte count falls below _____ cells/μL or if a category C AIDS indicator condition is present.

19. Macrophages serve as both targets and _____ for HIV.

20. During the _____ period, a person with HIV has few clinical manifestations but can transmit the infection to others.

UNIT III: Case Studies

Jane is a 12-year-old girl with a severe allergy to bee stings. She carries an emergency kit containing epinephrine with her at all times. The last time she was stung, she developed wheezing and severe urticaria.

1. Jane's sensitivity to bee stings is an example of
   A. type I hypersensitivity.
   B. type II hypersensitivity.
   C. type III hypersensitivity.
   D. type IV hypersensitivity.

2. Most of the signs and symptoms related to this type of hypersensitivity are attributable to
   A. activation of complement.
   B. release of inflammatory mediators from mast cells.
   C. excessive production of eosinophils.
   D. production of autoantibodies.

3. The purposes of the epinephrine injection include all of the following *except*
   A. stabilizing mast cell membranes.
   B. relaxing bronchial smooth muscle.
   C. supporting arterial blood pressure.
   D. blocking histamine receptors.

4. In addition to avoiding bee stings and immediately treating those that do occur with epinephrine, Jane might benefit from
   A. immunosuppressive therapy with steroids.
   B. desensitization therapy.
   C. plasmapheresis.
   D. cytotoxic therapy.

Stan is a 58-year-old man in the clinic for evaluation of back pain. He is sent for an x-ray film, which reveals multiple areas of reduced bone density and a compression fracture of a vertebra. His laboratory work demonstrates an elevated serum calcium level.

5. Which of the following diseases is most consistent with these findings?
   A. Leukemia
   B. Osteoporosis
   C. Plasma cell myeloma
   D. Lymphoma

6. Which of the following findings would help confirm this diagnosis?
   A. Elevated white blood cell count
   B. Monoclonal antibody spike on electrophoresis
   C. More than 30% blast cells in the bone marrow aspirant
   D. Reed-Sternberg cells in the biopsy sample

7. Stan undergoes a bone marrow biopsy the result of which reveals an abnormally high percentage of plasma cells. This means that his disease is a cancer of
   A. T cells.
   B. B cells.
   C. granulocytes.
   D. monocytes.

Ken is a 36-year-old man with a history of intravenous drug abuse. He was diagnosed as HIV positive 3 years ago and has been taking antiretroviral therapy since then. He has generally been well and comes to the clinic for checkups about every 3 months. At this visit his CD4 count is 198 cells/uL.

8. Testing demonstrates that Ken's viral load is below the level detected by the serum assay. This means that
   A. he is responding appropriately to therapy.
   B. his protease inhibitor can be discontinued.
   C. his HIV disease has been eliminated.
   D. his reverse transcriptase inhibitor can be discontinued.

9. The finding that Ken's CD4 lymphocyte count is 198 cells/µL means that
   A. he has less than a year to live.
   B. his diagnosis is changed from HIV disease to AIDS.
   C. he is unlikely to benefit from further therapy.
   D. he is no longer able to mount an immune response.

10. To avoid transmitting HIV to his girlfriend, Ken is taught to practice safe sex, which includes all of the following *except*
    A. abstinence.
    B. using condoms.
    C. using spermicidal ointments.
    D. maintaining a low viral load.

11. Ken's girlfriend may be a candidate for Prep, preexposure prophylaxis. This therapy is most appropriate for sexual partners who
    A. are HIV positive but have normal CD4 counts.
    B. are HIV negative but at high risk for exposure.
    C. are HIV negative but at low risk for exposure.
    D. are HIV positive and at high risk for AIDS.

13 Alterations in Oxygen Transport

MATCHING

Match each definition on the left with its term on the right. Not all terms are defined.

Definitions

1. _____ Not actually cells; fragments of megakaryocytes

2. _____ Cells found in the blood that are important in the inflammatory and immune responses

3. _____ A hormone produced by the kidney that is necessary for red blood cell (RBC) production.

4. _____ Average volume of blood in the circulatory system of an adult

5. _____ Major component of RBCs to which oxygen molecules bind

6. _____ Normal life span of RBCs

7. _____ Percentage of the blood that consists of cells

8. _____ Required for adequate synthesis of RBCs; absorbed intestinally associated with intrinsic factor

9. _____ Substance released during RBC degradation

10. _____ Mature blood cells that leave the bloodstream for the tissues, where they are powerful phagocytes

11. _____ Bone marrow cell from which all blood cells are derived

12. _____ Immature RBCs normally representing 1% of the RBC count

13. _____ A factor that influences the affinity of hemoglobin for oxygen

14. _____ Force that drives oxygen to bind to hemoglobin

15. _____ Amount of hemoglobin bound to oxygen compared with total amount of hemoglobin in the blood

Terms

A. Oxygen saturation
B. Bilirubin
C. Reticulocyte
D. Vitamin B_{12}
E. Hemoglobin
F. pH
G. Macrophages
H. Platelets
I. 45%
J. Partial pressure of O_2
K. Erythropoietin
L. 5 liters
M. Myeloid stem cell
N. Monocytes
O. Metabolic rate
P. Leukocytes
Q. Folate
R. Lymphoid stem cell
S. Iron
T. 80 to 120 days
U. Pluripotent stem cell
V. 55%

MULTIPLE CHOICE

Select the one best answer to each of the following questions.

16. Which of the following statements about the oxyhemoglobin dissociation curve is *true*?
    A. The curve shifts to the right with alkalosis.
    B. Hemoglobin levels of below normal will affect the curve.
    C. The curve shifts to the left with an increase in CO_2.
    D. Saturation is most affected when the Pao_2 falls below 60 mm Hg.

17. The pancytopenia associated with aplastic anemia may present with a variety of signs and symptoms, including
    A. bleeding.
    B. increased immune cell function.
    C. increased oxygen saturation levels.
    D. thrombocytosis.

18. Sickle cell crisis causes symptoms related to the anemia and
    A. vasospasms.
    B. vascular obstruction.
    C. increased risk of acute infection.
    D. bleeding.

19. Erythroblastosis fetalis (hemolytic disease of the newborn) occurs because
    A. the mother has taken medications that cause a decrease in the RBC life span.
    B. the mother and father differ in ABO blood type.
    C. Rh factor incompatibility results in antibody formation against fetal RBCs.
    D. maternal RBCs cross the placenta and stimulate antibody production.

20. The earliest clinical indicator of acute blood loss is
    A. absence of urine production.
    B. elevated heart rate at rest.
    C. postural hypotension.
    D. cold, clammy skin.

21. Secondary polycythemia would most likely develop in a patient
    A. who has chronic hypoxemia associated with chronic bronchitis.
    B. who has chronic bleeding associated with a gastric ulcer.
    C. who has dehydration associated with gastrointestinal flu.
    D. who is spending a weekend in the mountains.

22. The arterial oxygen content (CaO_2) for a patient with a PaO_2 of 75 mm Hg, an SaO_2 of 87%, and a hemoglobin level of 12 g/dL would be
    A. 13.9 mL oxygen/dL.
    B. 1421.5 mL oxygen/dL.
    C. 1399 mL oxygen/dL.
    D. 14.2 mL oxygen/dL.

FILL IN THE BLANKS

Fill in the blanks with the appropriate word or words.

23. Fill in the anemia table below with E (for elevated), N (for normal), or D (for decreased) for the mean corpuscular volume (MCV) and mean corpuscular hemoglobin concentration (MCHC).

Anemia Disorder	MCV	MCHC
Iron deficiency		
Aplastic		
Vitamin B_{12} deficiency		
Folate deficiency		
Thalassemia		
Hemolytic		
Acute blood loss		
Erythropoietin deficiency		

24. Mature erythrocytes have no organelles and must rely on _____ for cellular energy production.

25. When RBCs are degraded, the porphyrin component of hemoglobin is reduced to _____, which is poorly soluble in water and binds to albumin in the plasma.

26. When fully saturated, each gram of hemoglobin carries approximately _____ mL of oxygen.

27. The normal CaO_2 is about _____ mL of oxygen per deciliter and is calculated by the following formula:

$$CaO_2 = (\underline{\hspace{2cm}} \times 0.003) + (Hb \text{ g/dL} \times \underline{\hspace{2cm}} \times \underline{\hspace{2cm}}).$$

28. Under normal conditions, about _____ % of the oxygen carried in arterial blood is unloaded at the tissues.

29. The serum erythropoietin level can be helpful in differentiating polycythemia vera from secondary polycythemia because it is elevated in _____ _____ and low in _____ _____.

30. _____ is a breakdown byproduct of RBCs that is transported to the liver, where it is _____ and eliminated in bile.

14 Alterations in Hemostasis and Blood Coagulation

TRUE/FALSE

Indicate whether the following statements regarding hemostasis and coagulation disorders are true (T) or false (F).

1. _____ Antithrombin and protein C bind to and inhibit several activated clotting factors.

2. _____ A patient having excessive bleeding associated with aspirin use would have normal partial thromboplastin (PT)/international normalized ratio (INR) and activated partial thromboplastin time (aPTT) values but a prolonged bleeding time.

3. _____ The pinpoint skin spots associated with thrombocytopenia (petechiae) blanch when pressure is applied to them.

4. _____ A patient with a platelet count of 200,000/μL would be diagnosed with thrombocythemia.

5. _____ Tissue plasminogen activator stimulates the conversion of plasminogen to plasmin and increases fibrinolysis.

MULTIPLE CHOICE

Select the one best answer to each of the following questions.

6. Activation of the intrinsic pathway of coagulation is initiated by
   A. heparin.
   B. tissue thromboplastin.
   C. blood contact with injured vascular endothelium.
   D. factor X.

7. Fibrinolysis results in
   A. activation of the clotting cascade.
   B. conversion of plasminogen to plasmin.
   C. conversion of fibrinogen to fibrin.
   D. increased amounts of fibrin split products.

8. Deficient production of clotting factors would occur if which of the following organs were functioning poorly?
   A. Liver
   B. Kidneys
   C. Lungs
   D. Bone marrow

9. The proper function of the extrinsic pathway of coagulation is best measured by which of the following laboratory tests?
   A. PT/INR
   B. aPTT
   C. Platelet count
   D. Bleeding time

10. A common over-the-counter medication that can alter hemostasis is
    A. acetaminophen (Tylenol).
    B. antihistamine.
    C. multivitamins.
    D. ibuprofen (nonsteroidal antiinflammatory drug [NSAID]).

11. Vitamin K deficiency in an adult may be associated with
    A. overdosage of heparin.
    B. liver disease.
    C. gallbladder removal.
    D. ingestion of large quantities of green leafy vegetables.

12. Pathologic activation of the clotting cascade producing widespread coagulation and subsequent bleeding from a deficiency of clotting factors occurs in
    A. von Willebrand disease.
    B. disseminated intravascular coagulation (DIC).
    C. hemophilia A.
    D. hepatitis.

13. All of the following are true regarding *primary* hemostasis *except*
    A. platelets release aggregation factors.
    B. vasoconstriction reduces blood loss.
    C. platelets adhere to injured endothelial surfaces.
    D. fibrin is rapidly degraded.

14. The presence of a group of petechiae in a patch of skin is called
    A. ecchymosis.
    B. telangiectasia.
    C. purpura.
    D. epistaxis.

15. Which of the following statements regarding clotting factors is *true*?
    A. All clotting factors require the availability of vitamin K.
    B. Clotting factors are inactivated when outside the body.
    C. Low-molecular-weight heparins block function of all clotting factors.
    D. Most clotting factors circulate in inactive form.

FILL IN THE BLANKS

16. Fill in the hemostasis disorder table below with E (elevated or prolonged), N (normal), or D (decreased) for each laboratory finding.

Hemostasis Disorder	Platelet Count	PT/INR	aPTT	Bleeding Time
Idiopathic thrombocytopenic purpura				
Hemophilia A or B				
Liver disease				
Aspirin use				
DIC				

17. Platelets aggregate together by binding to fibrinogen with their _____ _____ receptors.

18. Aspirin and other NSAIDs inhibit platelet function by inhibiting the enzyme _____, which decreases the production of prostaglandins and thromboxanes.

19. The _____ pathway is activated by external traumatic injury of blood vessel walls, whereas the _____ pathway is activated by damaged endothelial walls.

20. _____ is the medical term for a bruise, and _____ means blood in the urine.

15 Alterations in Blood Flow

TRUE/FALSE

Indicate whether the following statements are true (T) or false (F).

1. _____ As with veins, lymphatic vessels have valves that prevent backflow and enhance forward movement.

2. _____ A cerebrovascular accident (stroke) is a serious complication of a thromboembolus leaving the right atrium.

3. _____ The greatest risk associated with aneurysms is rupture.

4. _____ A common cause of lymphedema is surgical removal of lymph nodes for breast cancer.

5. _____ Arteriosclerosis and atherosclerosis are synonymous terms.

6. _____ Normal resting cardiac output for an adult is approximately 5 L/min.

7. _____ The intimal layer of arteries contains large amounts of muscle.

8. _____ Capillary permeability normally is determined by the thickness of the basement membrane.

9. _____ Administration of calcium channel antagonists (blockers) results in dilation of arterioles.

10. _____ Binding of norepinephrine to alpha-1 receptors on vascular smooth muscle results in constriction of arterioles.

MULTIPLE CHOICE

Select the one best answer to each of the following questions.

11. Capillary permeability is greatest in the
    A. blood–brain barrier.
    B. extremities.
    C. heart.
    D. kidney glomeruli.

12. Flow through a blood vessel is primarily regulated by alteration of its
    A. length.
    B. wall thickness.
    C. radius.
    D. distending pressure.

13. Blood pressure is highest in the
    A. capillaries.
    B. pulmonary artery.
    C. vena cava.
    D. aorta.

14. A common cause of edema in children is
    A. decreased capillary hydrostatic fluid pressure.
    B. increased interstitial hydrostatic fluid pressure.
    C. decreased interstitial fluid colloid osmotic pressure.
    D. decreased plasma colloid osmotic pressure.

44

15. Stimulation of the sympathetic nervous system causes constriction of
    A. bronchioles.
    B. arterioles.
    C. capillaries.
    D. lymphatics.

16. Which one of the following vessels has the most rapid blood flow (velocity)?
    A. Vena cava
    B. Capillaries
    C. Venules
    D. Arterioles

17. The ability of tissues to maintain local perfusion regardless of systemic arterial pressure is called
    A. hyperemia.
    B. vascular resistance.
    C. autoregulation.
    D. compensation.

18. Thrombus formation in the arterial system may produce
    A. ischemia.
    B. thrombophlebitis.
    C. edema.
    D. infection.

19. A risk factor enhancing the development of atherosclerosis is
    A. an increased level of high-density lipoproteins (HDLs).
    B. eating a high-protein diet.
    C. an elevated level of low-density lipoprotein (LDL) cholesterol.
    D. chronic low blood pressure.

20. The "six P's" associated with an acute arterial occlusion include all of the following *except*
    A. pallor.
    B. piloerection.
    C. pulselessness.
    D. pain.

21. The most common cause of pulmonary embolism is
    A. deep vein thrombosis.
    B. varicose veins.
    C. atherosclerosis.
    D. anemia.

22. The vasospastic arteriolar disorder that causes acute ischemic pain in hands or feet is called
    A. compartment syndrome.
    B. atherosclerosis.
    C. Buerger disease.
    D. Raynaud syndrome.

FILL IN THE BLANKS

Fill in the blanks with the appropriate word or words.

23. According to Ohm's law (Q = P/R), an increase in resistance (R) will result in a(n) _____ in flow (Q), and an increase in driving pressure (P) will result in a(n) _____ in flow.

24. Driving pressure is calculated by subtracting the pressure at the distal end of a tube (P2) from the pressure at the proximal end (P1). If the mean arterial pressure (MAP) is 80 mm Hg and the right atrial pressure (RAP) is 20 mm Hg, then the driving pressure through the systemic vessels is _____ mm Hg.

45

25. An increase in MAP will _____ driving pressure, whereas an increase in RAP will _____ driving pressure.

26. According to Poiseuille's law ($R = 8\,nl/\pi r^4$), a twofold increase in vessel radius (r) will result in a _____-fold reduction in resistance (R).

27. A twofold increase in vessel length (l) will result in a _____-fold increase in resistance (R).

28. Using the law of Laplace, name three conditions that would increase wall tension:

    1. _____

    2. _____

    3. _____

29. Calculate the capillary filtration pressure (mm Hg) if the capillary hydrostatic pressure is 40 mm Hg, capillary oncotic pressure is 35 mm Hg, tissue hydrostatic pressure is 2 mm Hg, and tissue oncotic pressure is zero:

    _____.

30. A tissue can increase its rate of blood flow by reducing its arteriolar _____.

16 Alterations in Blood Pressure

TRUE/FALSE

Indicate whether the following statements are true (T) or false (F).

1. _____ The goal level for antihypertensive therapy in all patients is less than 140/90 mm Hg.

2. _____ Systemic blood vessels are not significantly affected by parasympathetic innervation.

3. _____ The major determinant of systemic vascular resistance is the diameter of arterioles.

4. _____ Stimulation of the renin–angiotensin system results in a lowering of the mean arterial pressure (MAP).

5. _____ The primary reason blood pressure increases with age is because the heart becomes a less efficient pump.

6. _____ Blood pressure in the pulmonary vascular bed is higher than that in the systemic vascular bed.

7. _____ Systolic blood pressure measured at the dorsalis pedis artery in the foot should be the same or higher than the systolic pressure measured at the brachial artery.

8. _____ The pulse pressure for a patient with a blood pressure of 155/85 mm Hg would be 70 mm Hg.

9. _____ Normal blood pressure values are based on the patient lying supine.

10. _____ Standards of expected blood pressure differ depending on gender.

MULTIPLE CHOICE

Select the one best answer to each of the following questions.

11. The MAP for a patient with a blood pressure of 150/90 mm Hg would be
    A. 210 mm Hg.
    B. 80 mm Hg.
    C. 130 mm Hg.
    D. 110 mm Hg.

12. Stimulation of the baroreceptors in the carotid sinus and aortic arch due to increased blood pressure produces
    A. increased release of norepinephrine.
    B. increased MAP.
    C. increased cardiac output.
    D. increased parasympathetic inhibition of the heart rate.

13. Atrial natriuretic peptide
    A. is released from the atria in response to decreased preload.
    B. stimulates the release of renin, aldosterone, and antidiuretic hormone.
    C. increases excretion of water and sodium by the kidney.
    D. decreases the glomerular filtration rate.

14. Risk factors for hypertension include
    A. obesity.
    B. male gender.
    C. white race.
    D. moderate alcohol consumption.

15. A common cause of secondary hypertension is
   A. anemia.
   B. renal disease.
   C. myocardial infarction.
   D. dissecting aneurysm.

16. The stage of prehypertension is initially most appropriately managed with all of the following *except*
   A. exercise.
   B. dietary management.
   C. drug therapy.
   D. weight loss.

17. Orthostatic or postural hypotension would be present if a patient has a supine blood pressure of 118/75 mm Hg with a heart rate of 90 beats/min and if the following values are obtained when the patient's head is elevated to 90 degrees:
   A. Blood pressure 112/85 mm Hg, heart rate 98 beats/min.
   B. Blood pressure 110/80 mm Hg, heart rate 95 beats/min.
   C. Blood pressure 115/70 mm Hg, heart rate 100 beats/min.
   D. Blood pressure 110/75 mm Hg, heart rate 110 beats/min.

18. A patient with a blood pressure of 180/128 mm Hg and experiencing chest pain is categorized as having
   A. a hypertensive emergency.
   B. a hypertensive urgency.
   C. hypertension stage 1.
   D. hypertension stage 2.

FILL IN THE BLANKS

Fill in the blanks with the appropriate word or words.

19. Fill in the blood pressure ranges for each category of blood pressure in the table below using JNC-7 criteria (not changed in JNC-8).

Category	Systolic (mm Hg)	Diastolic (mm Hg)
Normal		
Prehypertension		
Hypertension, stage 1		
Hypertension, stage 2		

20. According to the American Heart Association, there are specific risk factors for atherosclerosis. List some of the modifiable and nonmodifiable risks below:

Modifiable	Nonmodifiable

21. Errors in the measurement of blood pressure have predictable effects. Note the likely effect for each error in the table below:

Error	Effect on Blood Pressure
Blood pressure cuff too large	
Arm positioned above heart	
Arm unsupported	
Less than 1 minute between readings	

22. When assessing blood pressure in children, a reading that is lower than the _____ th percentile for age and gender is considered normal.

23. Stage ___ hypertension is diagnosed when the systolic blood pressure is below 140 mm Hg but the diastolic pressure remains above _____ mm Hg.

24. When discussing the potential complications of poorly controlled hypertension with a patient, three important organ systems should be mentioned and assessed: _____, _____, and _____.

25. Pharmacologic interventions for hypertension affect one or more of the variables responsible for blood pressure. These are divided into three groups: drugs that reduce _____, _____, and _____.

UNIT IV: Case Studies

K.T. is a 25-year-old woman who came to the clinic complaining of increasing fatigue during the past few months and a recent onset (this week) of dyspnea and shortness of breath. A diagnosis of anemia is made when her laboratory results indicate a decreased red blood cell (RBC) count, decreased hemoglobin, and decreased RBC indices (mean corpuscular volume [MCV], mean corpuscular hemoglobin concentration [MCHC], and mean corpuscular hemoglobin [MCH]).

1. Based on these laboratory values, what type of anemia does K.T. likely have?
   A. Aplastic anemia
   B. Vitamin B_{12} deficiency anemia
   C. Folate deficiency anemia
   D. Iron deficiency anemia

2. The signs and symptoms of anemia are all related to what common pathophysiologic feature of the condition?
   A. Increased oxygen consumption by tissues
   B. Decreased blood oxygen content
   C. Vasodilation
   D. A shift in the oxyhemoglobin dissociation curve

3. A possible cause of K.T.'s anemia is
   A. bone marrow suppression.
   B. insufficient production of erythropoietin.
   C. autoimmune disease.
   D. chronic excessive blood loss during menstruation.

4. K.T. is prescribed an iron supplement and reevaluated in 3 months. Which of the following laboratory results would indicate that therapy is effective?
   A. Increased reticulocyte count
   B. Elevated total iron-binding capacity (TIBC)
   C. Elevated red cell distribution width (RDW)
   D. Increased iron level

49

Prolonged bleeding following a circumcision prompted an evaluation of J.K. for a disorder of hemostasis. Ultimately, he was diagnosed with hemophilia A.

5. Which of the following is true regarding hemophilia A?
   A. It is also known as Christmas disease.
   B. It is most often an X-linked disease.
   C. There is a deficiency of factor IX.
   D. There is an autosomal-dominant disorder of factor VIII.

6. Even when he is older, which of the following medications is contraindicated for J.K. because of his diagnosis?
   A. Antibiotics
   B. Calcium supplements
   C. Acetaminophen
   D. Aspirin

7. As J.K. begins to become more active, he will be at risk for the hallmark finding associated with hemophilia, which is
   A. hemarthrosis.
   B. purpura.
   C. anemia.
   D. telangiectasia.

8. Which of the following laboratory test results would be characteristic of hemophilia?
   A. Elevated factor VIII level
   B. Reduced platelet count
   C. Elevated prothrombin time (PT/INR)
   D. Elevated activated partial thromboplastin time (aPTT)

F.G. is being treated for chronic idiopathic thrombocytopenic purpura.

9. The underlying mechanism of this condition is
   A. aplastic anemia.
   B. failure of the liver to produce adequate numbers of platelets.
   C. unknown; it is possibly autoimmune.
   D. aspirin toxicity.

10. F.G., like other patients with this condition, presents with all of the following *except*
    A. decreased hemoglobin.
    B. ecchymosis.
    C. petechiae.
    D. hematomas.

11. Laboratory test results indicative of thrombocytopenia, in addition to a low platelet count, would be
    A. an increased PT/INR.
    B. a prolonged bleeding time and poor clot retraction.
    C. an increased aPTT.
    D. a decreased RBC count.

Because S.M. had a heart attack 2 months ago, he and his wife are very motivated to make the necessary lifestyle changes to reduce his risk of having another one. The nurse is working with this couple to reduce his risk factors for atherosclerosis.

12. S.M. is encouraged to raise his HDL levels as a protection against atherosclerosis. The goal for HDL levels should be
    A. less than 200 mg/dL.
    B. greater than 40 mg/dL.
    C. greater than 160 mg/dL.
    D. less than 35 mg/dL.

13. In addition to raising his HDL, S.M. is encouraged to lower his risk by taking a statin medication. In addition to lowering LDL, statins are thought to help by
    A. reducing serum glucose levels.
    B. reducing absorption of lipid from the gastrointestinal tract.
    C. reducing serum platelet levels.
    D. reducing inflammation in arterial walls.

14. Suggested dietary modifications for S.M. should include
    A. avoidance of hydrogenated and trans fatty acids and oils.
    B. use of only natural fats, such as those from animals and corn oil.
    C. use of sources of simple sugars to substitute for fat calories.
    D. use of stimulant dietary aids to achieve weight loss.

As part of his routine physical examination, G.H. had his blood pressure checked. It was found to be 170/100 mm Hg. G.H. is 54 years old, 5 feet 10 inches tall, and weighs 230 pounds. He is a commercial realtor. His serum cholesterol level is 265 mg/dL, his LDL level is 170 mg/dL, and his HDL level is 24 mg/dL. His father died after a second heart attack, and his mother had a stroke when she was 72; she is now living in a retirement community.

15. G.H. is asked to have his blood pressure measured again to verify that it is still elevated. This is done because
    A. numerous factors can cause spurious blood pressure elevations.
    B. it is unlikely that his blood pressure is really this high.
    C. everyone experiences "white coat" phenomenon during a physical examination.
    D. no treatment is indicated for a blood pressure of 170/100 mm Hg.

16. Which of the following statements regarding G.H.'s hypertension diagnosis is *true*?
    A. His only risk factors are modifiable ones.
    B. Lifestyle modifications should be sufficient treatment.
    C. His hypertension is classified as secondary.
    D. He has stage 2 hypertension.

17. G.H. is not enthusiastic about having treatment for his hypertension. "But I really feel fine," he tells the nurse. The nurse explains that therapy should be initiated immediately because
    A. management of elevated blood pressure now will solve the problem, after which therapy can be stopped.
    B. elevated blood pressure causes organ damage before signs or symptoms are evident.
    C. aggressive management of hypertension will prevent a heart attack or stroke.
    D. if the hypertension is not managed now, it will continue to elevate.

P.R. is 24 years old and 6 months pregnant with her first child. She has had a normal pregnancy to this point, but during this visit her blood pressure is found to have increased from her previous baseline of 116/74 mm Hg to 150/98 mm Hg. Her nurse practitioner suspects preeclampsia (pregnancy-induced hypertension).

18. In addition to hypertension, preeclampsia is characterized by
    A. nausea and vomiting.
    B. fatigue and lower back pain.
    C. protein in the urine and edema.
    D. retinal changes and rales in the lungs.

19. Three months after delivery of the baby, P.R.'s blood pressure remains elevated at 150/98 mm Hg. A thorough workup reveals no identifiable cause for the high blood pressure, and a diagnosis of

    _____ is made.
    A. chronic preeclampsia
    B. postpartum hypertension
    C. secondary hypertension
    D. primary, or essential, hypertension

20. Normally, blood pressure falls slightly during the first 6 months of pregnancy. This is caused by
    A. decreased systemic vascular resistance.
    B. increased cardiac output.
    C. decreased heart rate.
    D. decreased circulating blood volume.

17 Cardiac Function

MATCHING

1. Match each of the following anatomic terms with the appropriate letter in the figure.

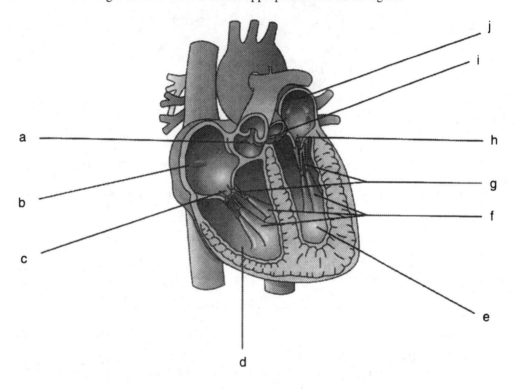

_____ Pulmonary valve   _____ Left atrium

_____ Tricuspid valve   _____ Aortic valve

_____ Right atrium   _____ Mitral valve

_____ Right ventricle   _____ Chordae tendineae

_____ Left ventricle   _____ Papillary muscles

2. Match each of the following anatomic terms with the appropriate letter in the figure.

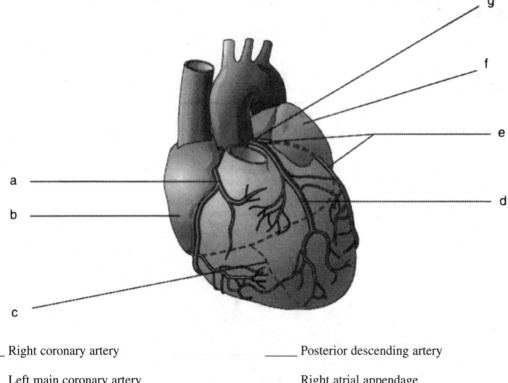

_____ Right coronary artery   _____ Posterior descending artery

_____ Left main coronary artery   _____ Right atrial appendage

_____ Left circumflex artery   _____ Left atrial appendage

_____ Left anterior descending artery

TRUE/FALSE

Indicate whether the following statements regarding the anatomy and physiology of the cardiac system are true (T) or false (F).

3. _____ The right atrium and ventricle form the anterior portion of the heart.

4. _____ The point of maximal impulse is normally located at the intersection of the fifth intercostal space and the left midclavicular line.

5. _____ The mitral valve is located between the right atrium and the right ventricle.

6. _____ The pulmonic and aortic valves usually have two cusps (bicuspid).

7. _____ Chordae tendineae tether the aortic and pulmonic valves to the myocardium.

8. _____ Left ventricular muscle is two to three times thicker than the right ventricular muscle.

9. _____ The endocardium is the inner surface of the heart chambers.

10. _____ Visceral pericardium is attached to the epicardial surface of the heart.

11. _____ Blood in the pulmonary veins is normally well oxygenated.

12. _____ The left atrium receives blood from the pulmonary artery.

13. _____ The left coronary artery perfuses the posterior aspect of the left ventricle in most individuals.

14. _____ Normally, the principal determinant of coronary artery resistance is coronary artery radius.

15. _____ The coronary arteries originate in the aorta, just distal to the aortic valve.

16. _____ Most blood flow through the coronary arteries occurs during ventricular systole.

17. _____ The left coronary artery has two principal branches, the left circumflex and the left anterior descending branches.

LABELING

18. Label the appropriate part of the figure with each of the following cardiac cycle events:

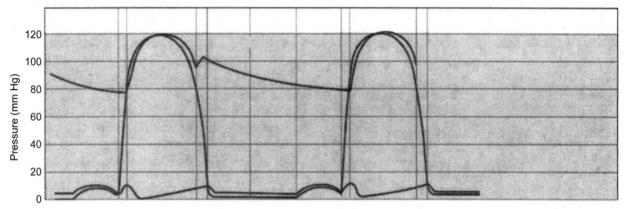

A wave	Aortic valve closure
C wave	Aortic valve opening
V wave	Dicrotic notch
Ventricular diastole	Isovolumic contraction
Ventricular ejection	Isovolumic relaxation
Time of S_1	Atrial systole
Time of S_2	

19. Describe the ionic events during each of the five phases of the cardiac action potential shown in the figure:

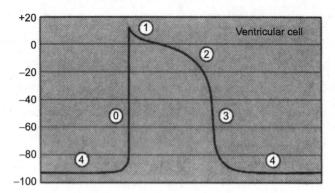

Phase 0:

Phase 1:

Phase 2:

Phase 3:

Phase 4:

MULTIPLE CHOICE

Select the one best answer to each of the following questions.

20. The myocardial cells of the heart contract synchronously as a syncytium because
    A. they are connected by gap junctions.
    B. they have one continuous cell membrane.
    C. they are all innervated by the same neuron.
    D. they all have the same rate of spontaneous depolarization.

21. The proteins that make up the contractile apparatus of a myocardial cell include all of the following *except*
    A. troponin.
    B. tropomyosin.
    C. actin.
    D. myoglobin.

22. Contraction of cardiac muscle is initiated by
    A. adenosine triphosphate (ATP) hydrolysis by myosin head groups.
    B. an increase in free intracellular calcium ion concentration.
    C. opening of voltage-gated potassium channels.
    D. binding of troponin and tropomyosin.

23. The affinity of myosin head groups for binding actin is decreased when myosin binds
    A. ATP.
    B. GTP.
    C. ADP.
    D. calcium.

24. Relaxation of cardiac muscle is an energy-requiring process because energy is needed
    A. for the sodium–potassium pump.
    B. to break actin–myosin cross-bridges.
    C. to pump calcium ions out of the cytosol.
    D. to close voltage-gated sodium channels.

25. Creatine phosphate
    A. is a marker of cardiac cell death.
    B. can donate a high-energy phosphate to adenosine diphosphate (ADP) to form ATP.
    C. is stored in large quantities in most cells.
    D. has different isoforms in different cell types.

26. Which of the following statements about the ventricular myocardial action potential is *not* correct?
    A. Fast voltage-gated sodium ion channels are open during phase 0.
    B. Slow voltage-gated calcium channels are open during phase 2.
    C. Repolarization is accomplished by the Na^+/K^+ pump during phase 3.
    D. Voltage-gated potassium channels are open during phases 1, 2, and 3.

27. Pacemaker cells can generate action potentials because
    A. they are hyperpolarized at rest.
    B. they have receptors for autonomic neurotransmitters.
    C. they spontaneously open cation (Na^+, Ca^{2+}) channels during phase 4.
    D. they spontaneously open chloride channels during phase 4.

28. Sympathetic nervous system action on pacemaker cells
    A. increases chloride ion flow across the cell membrane.
    B. increases potassium ion efflux across the cell membrane.
    C. decreases sodium ion influx across the cell membrane.
    D. increases calcium ion influx across the cell membrane.

29. Parasympathetic nervous system action on pacemaker cells
    A. increases calcium ion conductance across the cell membrane.
    B. increases potassium ion conductance across the cell membrane.
    C. increases sodium ion conductance across the cell membrane.
    D. decreases chloride ion conductance across the cell membrane.

30. The usual sequence of depolarization of the ventricles begins with
    A. right ventricular muscle.
    B. septal muscle.
    C. left ventricular apex muscle.
    D. the lateral wall of the left ventricle.

31. The PR interval of the electrocardiogram corresponds to depolarization of
    A. the atria.
    B. the AV node.
    C. the atria, AV node, and His-Purkinje fibers.
    D. the ventricular septum.

32. Cardiac output is the product of heart rate and
    A. contractility.
    B. blood pressure.
    C. stroke volume.
    D. preload.

33. Which of the following would result in a decrease in cardiac output?
    A. Increased preload
    B. Increased contractility
    C. Increased afterload
    D. Increased heart rate

34. Contractility is enhanced by factors that increase
    A. parasympathetic activity.
    B. stroke volume.
    C. baroreceptor activity.
    D. intracellular free calcium ions.

35. The Frank-Starling law of the heart suggests that increased preload will
    A. decrease cardiac workload.
    B. increase cardiac heart rate.
    C. increase stroke volume.
    D. increase afterload.

18 Alterations in Cardiac Function

COMPARE/CONTRAST

1. *Compare and contrast myocardial infarction (MI) and stable angina by filling in the table.*

Characteristic	MI	Stable Angina Pectoris
Pain character		
Electrocardiographic findings		
Serum marker elevations		

MULTIPLE CHOICE

Select the one best answer to each of the following questions.

2. The most common cause of cardiac ischemia is
   A. hypoxemia.
   B. excessive myocardial oxygen demand.
   C. anemia.
   D. reduced coronary artery blood flow.

3. Ischemic heart disease is nearly always a consequence of
   A. atherosclerosis.
   B. dysrhythmias.
   C. primary cardiomyopathies.
   D. myocarditis.

4. Which property of coronary lesions is thought to be most susceptible to acute occlusion?
   A. Fatty streak
   B. Large lipid core
   C. Thick fibrous cap
   D. Calcified plaque

5. Chronic partial occlusion of a coronary artery is associated with the clinical syndrome of
   A. unstable angina.
   B. stable angina.
   C. MI.
   D. Acute coronary syndrome.

6. The clinical syndromes of coronary heart disease include all of the following *except*
   A. stable angina pectoris.
   B. MI.
   C. chronic ischemic cardiomyopathy.
   D. myocarditis.

7. Stable angina pectoris
   A. results in permanent myocardial cell damage.
   B. is detected by elevated serum marker proteins.
   C. is usually relieved by rest.
   D. rarely lasts longer than 3 seconds.

8. Which of the following is considered the least specific serum indicator of myocardial cell death?
   A. Myoglobin
   B. Troponin I
   C. Creatine kinase, myocardial band (CK-MB)
   D. Troponin T

9. Ongoing acute cardiac ischemia is indicated on the ECG by
   A. abnormally large Q waves.
   B. abnormally small R waves.
   C. ST-segment elevation.
   D. inverted P waves.

10. The compensatory responses that are triggered following MI serve to
    A. protect the heart from damage.
    B. maintain cardiac output.
    C. reduce myocardial oxygen consumption.
    D. reduce cardiac workload.

11. The objectives of immediate treatment for acute coronary syndrome are to improve coronary perfusion and to
    A. reduce myocardial oxygen demand.
    B. reverse the atherosclerotic process.
    C. remove all potential risk factors.
    D. begin antilipid therapy.

12. Stenosis of a cardiac valve results in
    A. a back flow of blood through the valve.
    B. extra "volume" work for the heart.
    C. a pressure gradient across the valve when open.
    D. a bounding pulse.

13. The murmur of aortic stenosis
    A. occurs during ventricular diastole.
    B. is heard best at the apex.
    C. radiates to the neck.
    D. obliterates S_1 and S_2.

14. Mitral regurgitation
    A. results in large left atrial V waves on the atrial pressure monitor.
    B. produces a diastolic murmur.
    C. increases left ventricular afterload.
    D. produces a pressure gradient across the mitral valve during diastole.

15. Bacterial endocarditis most commonly affects valves
    A. on the left side of the heart.
    B. that are structurally abnormal.
    C. of elderly individuals.
    D. of patients with ischemic cardiomyopathy.

16. Myocarditis is an inflammatory disorder that
    A. is most commonly associated with streptococcal infections.
    B. often leads to dilated cardiomyopathy.
    C. results in hypertrophy of all four chambers of the heart.
    D. impairs left ventricular filling.

17. Cardiac tamponade compresses the heart chambers and produces
    A. arterial hypertension.
    B. accentuated heart sounds.
    C. adventitious heart sounds (S_3, S_4).
    D. pulsus paradoxus.

18. Which of the following findings is most indicative of pericarditis?
    A. Hypotension
    B. Pericardial friction rub
    C. Bounding pulse
    D. Displaced point of maximal impulse

19. Acyanotic congenital heart defects include
    A. tetralogy of Fallot.
    B. transposition of the great vessels.
    C. truncus arteriosus.
    D. patent ductus arteriosus.

20. Congenital heart defects that produce left-to-right shunts
    A. cause systemic hypoxemia.
    B. increase right ventricular workload.
    C. are cyanotic lesions.
    D. are without consequence.

FILL IN THE BLANKS

Fill in the blanks with the appropriate word or words.

21. Important characteristics of vulnerable coronary plaques are exposure to high shear stress, inflammation, _____

    _____ _____, and _____ _____.

22. Five syndromes of coronary heart disease can be differentiated. These include two chronic presentations, _____

    and _____, and three acute presentations, _____, _____, and

    _____. In practice, MI and unstable angina are similar at the onset, and the term _____

    is applied to both.

23. The risk of sustaining a coronary event is higher in those with elevated high-sensitivity C-reactive protein levels,

    indicating that _____ is an important etiologic factor for coronary heart disease.

24. A patient who presents at the emergency department with chest pain and ST elevation on the ECG is a candidate for

    _____ therapy.

25. A patient who presents at the emergency department with acute coronary syndrome and ST elevation that progresses
    to MI is diagnosed with ST elevation MI (STEMI), whereas a similar patient whose ST elevation does not progress

    to MI is diagnosed with _____ _____.

26. A patient who does not have ST elevation on the ECG but still suffers an acute MI as evidenced by elevated serum

    cardiac enzymes is diagnosed with _____.

27. A patient who is exhibiting signs and symptoms of acute coronary syndrome should be directed to take a(n)

    _____ orally immediately.

28. Rheumatic heart disease and rheumatic fever are uncommon but severe consequences of infection with

_____ _____ _____ _____.

29. Individuals who experience rheumatic fever have a _____ % chance of recurrence if they are reinfected and should receive chronic prophylactic antibiotic therapy.

30. In North America, most cases of myocarditis are thought to be a consequence of _____ infections; however, the infective organism is rarely identified.

31. Defects in the structure of myocardial _____ proteins are thought to cause most forms of hypertrophic cardiomyopathy.

32. Pathologic Q waves on an ECG occur because cells that are completely _____ are incapable of

_____ activity.

33. Three nonmodifiable risk factors for coronary artery disease are _____, _____, and

_____ _____.

34. High levels of _____ cholesterol may protect against atherosclerosis, whereas high levels of

_____ cholesterol may contribute to atherosclerosis risk.

35. A person who sustains a lateral wall MI likely had an occlusion of the _____ _____ coronary artery.

19 Heart Failure and Dysrhythmias: Common Sequelae of Cardiac Diseases

MULTIPLE CHOICE

Select the one best answer to each of the following questions.

1. Heart failure has occurred when
   A. the cardiac output falls below 5 L/min.
   B. a myocardial infarction (MI) destroys more than 20% of the heart muscle.
   C. a high workload is imposed on the heart.
   D. the cardiac output is insufficient to meet the demands of organs and tissues.

2. The most common underlying cause of heart failure is
   A. hypertension.
   B. coronary heart disease.
   C. hypertrophic cardiomyopathy.
   D. valvular dysfunction.

3. Patients with heart failure with preserved ejection fraction (EF) have symptoms of heart failure, but
   A. the cardiac output is normal.
   B. the ejection fraction is greater than 0.50.
   C. there is no edema formation.
   D. they are volume depleted.

4. Backward effects of isolated left-sided heart failure include
   A. pulmonary vascular congestion.
   B. jugular vein distention.
   C. dependent edema in the legs.
   D. bounding pulses.

5. Left-sided heart failure may lead to right-sided heart failure because of
   A. excessive volume retention.
   B. poor perfusion of the right coronary artery.
   C. increased right ventricular afterload.
   D. arterial hypotension.

6. Most patients with heart failure need medications to
   A. reduce afterload.
   B. increase contractility.
   C. reduce preload.
   D. reduce heart rate.

7. Which of these drug classes is contraindicated for most patients with heart failure because it is associated with a higher mortality risk?
   A. Diuretic agents
   B. β-receptor blockers
   C. Angiotensin-converting enzyme (ACE) inhibitors
   D. Positive inotropic agents

8. Which of the following agents have been shown to reduce mortality in patients with systolic heart failure?
   A. Loop diuretics
   B. Inotropic agents (β_1-agonists, digitalis)
   C. ACE inhibitors and β-blockers
   D. Calcium channel blockers

9. Backward effects of right-sided heart failure include
   A. jugular venous distention.
   B. cough.
   C. increased heart rate.
   D. rales in the lung bases.

10. All of the following are characteristics of normal sinus rhythm *except*
    A. a PR interval of 0.12 to 0.20 second.
    B. one P wave for each QRS complex.
    C. a rate of 60 to 100 beats/min.
    D. a QRS duration of 0.4 to 0.6 second.

11. Which of the following dysrhythmias is attributed to reentry mechanism?
    A. Ventricular fibrillation
    B. Asystole
    C. Sinus bradycardia
    D. Junctional escape rhythm

12. A first-degree conduction block is characterized by
    A. bradycardia.
    B. dropped P waves.
    C. a prolonged PR interval.
    D. a widened QRS complex.

13. Type 1 (Wenckebach/Mobitz I) second-degree block is characterized by
    A. dropped P waves with a consistent PR interval.
    B. no apparent association between P waves and QRS complexes.
    C. progressive lengthening of the PR interval until a P wave is not conducted.
    D. bizarre-looking QRS complexes.

14. The most important consideration in determining treatment for dysrhythmias is
    A. how frequently they occur.
    B. whether they are causing symptoms.
    C. the underlying disease process.
    D. how bizarre the complexes appear.

15. Sinus tachycardia is associated with all of the following *except*
    A. a prolonged PR interval.
    B. a heart rate greater than 100 beats/min in adults.
    C. a normal response to acute pain and fever.
    D. a normal QRS interval.

TRUE/FALSE

Indicate whether the following statements regarding heart failure or dysrhythmias are true (T) or false (F).

16. _____ The patient with only diastolic heart failure has a near normal ejection fraction.

17. _____ Myocardial hypertrophy is associated with an increased overall number of cardiac muscle cells.

18. _____ Forward effects of heart failure occur because of reduced perfusion of the brain and other peripheral organ systems.

19. _____ The New York Heart Association classes categorize heart failure patients by structural indicators and clinical symptoms.

20. _____ Physiologic compensations activated in heart failure reduce progression of the disease.

21. _____ Abnormal automaticity is often caused by hypokalemia.

22. _____ Digitalis toxicity and excessive sympathetic stimulation may cause dysrhythmias due to delayed afterdepolarization.

23. _____ The heart rate on an ECG is most accurately determined by counting the number of QRS complexes in a 6-second strip, then multiplying by 10.

24. _____ No P waves are seen on an ECG strip of a junctional dysrhythmia.

25. _____ Electrical *asystole* means complete absence of electrical activity.

Match the rhythm strip on the right with its correct interpretation on the left.

26. _____ Premature ventricular complex

27. _____ Atrial fibrillation

28. _____ Premature atrial complex

29. _____ Type I Wenckebach block

30. _____ Ventricular tachycardia

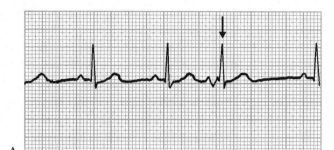

A.

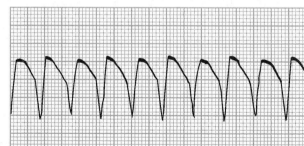

B.

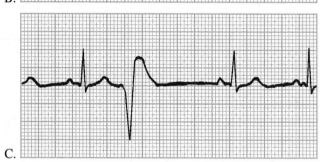

C.

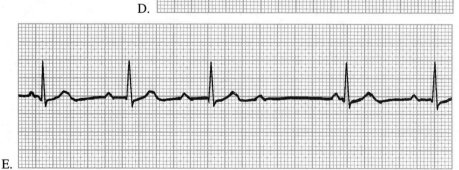

D.

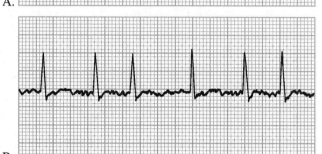

E.

Chapter **19 Heart Failure and Dysrhythmias: Common Sequelae of Cardiac Diseases**

20 Shock

MATCHING

Match the etiology on the left with the type of shock on the right. Answers may be used more than once.

1. _____ Prolonged vomiting or diarrhea
2. _____ Severe allergy to peanuts
3. _____ Spinal cord injury
4. _____ End-stage heart failure
5. _____ Burns
6. _____ Overwhelming infection
7. _____ Acute blood loss
8. _____ Spinal anesthesia

A. Anaphylactic
B. Cardiogenic
C. Hypovolemic
D. Neurogenic
E. Septic

MULTIPLE CHOICE

Select the one best answer to each of the following questions.

9. The common finding in all types of circulatory shock is
   A. low blood volume.
   B. low cardiac output.
   C. poor prognosis.
   D. cellular hypoxia.

10. In the early compensated stage of circulatory shock, blood pressure is maintained because of
    A. increased cardiac output.
    B. increased systemic vascular resistance.
    C. increased preload.
    D. venoconstriction.

11. An increased serum lactate level (lactic acidosis) is commonly used as a marker of
    A. cell death.
    B. anaerobic metabolism.
    C. inflammation.
    D. early shock.

12. A reduced oxygen extraction rate as indicated by a high systemic venous oxygen saturation is associated with
    A. cardiogenic shock.
    B. hypovolemic shock.
    C. neurogenic shock.
    D. septic shock.

13. Types of shock categorized by abnormal distribution of cardiac output (distributive shock) include all of the following, *except*
    A. hypovolemic shock.
    B. septic shock.
    C. anaphylactic shock.
    D. neurogenic shock.

67

14. Septic shock is characterized by an abnormally low systemic vascular resistance because of
    A. high cardiac output.
    B. cytokine-induced production of nitric oxide.
    C. sympathetic nervous system dysfunction.
    D. widespread release of histamine.

15. The physiologic responses occurring in compensatory shock are primarily from
    A. release of antidiuretic hormone.
    B. myocardial depressant factor.
    C. activation of the sympathetic nervous system.
    D. initiation of the coagulation cascade.

FILL IN THE BLANKS

Fill in the blanks with the appropriate word or words.

16. The immune system propagates further tissue damage in the _____ stage of shock.

17. Hemodynamic monitoring allows the assessment of the adequacy of cardiac output in an individual, called the _____ _____, which is cardiac output adjusted for the patient's size.

18. In cardiogenic shock, compensatory mechanisms, working via the RAAS, increase cardiac _____ and therefore _____.

19. In the adult, hemorrhagic hypovolemic shock is classified as moderate if the loss is _____ to _____ mL.

20. Dextran, albumin, and hetastarch are classified as _____.

21. Septic shock is often associated with infection with gram-negative bacteria because of their release of _____.

22. Anaphylactic shock is most frequently caused by a type _____ hypersensitivity reaction, which involves _____ antibodies.

23. Acute renal failure is a potential complication of shock due to _____ perfusion, producing _____ tubule cells.

24. Mortality rates are lowest for _____ shock and highest for _____ shock.

25. In the stage of refractory shock, patients are _____ to treatment interventions.

UNIT V: Case Studies

P.J. is a 67-year-old man with a long history of stable angina who is treated with nitroglycerin tablets as needed for chest pain. He has mild hypertension, which is well controlled by diet and an angiotensin-converting enzyme (ACE) inhibitor.

1. P.J. has noticed that his chest pain is occurring with increasing frequency, and less activity is required to initiate the symptoms; however, the pain subsides quickly with rest and one or two nitroglycerin tablets. These symptoms are consistent with a diagnosis of
   A. stable angina.
   B. progressive angina.
   C. unstable angina.
   D. variant angina.

2. P.J. should be counseled to seek medical care immediately when
   A. chest pain occurs more than three to five times per week.
   B. mild shortness of breath accompanies the chest pain.
   C. chest pain is not relieved within 5 minutes.
   D. chest pain occurs at rest or is not relieved within 15 minutes.

3. Effective control of P.J.'s blood pressure is important for all of the following reasons, *except*
   A. high blood pressure is a risk factor for atherosclerosis.
   B. high blood pressure increases the left ventricular afterload.
   C. high blood pressure reduces the coronary artery perfusion pressure.
   D. high blood pressure contributes to the development of left ventricular hypertrophy.

4. One morning at about 4:00 AM, P.J. is awakened from sleep with chest pain and shortness of breath. The pain is much more severe than his usual anginal pain and radiates to the jaw and left arm. He is diaphoretic and pale. His wife calls for emergency assistance, and P.J. is transported to the local emergency department. Upon admission, the ECG shows significant ST-segment elevation, which indicates
   A. acute coronary syndrome.
   B. impending dysrhythmia.
   C. recent myocardial infarction (MI).
   D. cardiac irritation.

5. The ST elevation is noted only in leads II, III, and aVF, indicating that the affected area of the heart is the
   A. right ventricle.
   B. intraventricular septum.
   C. anterolateral wall of the left ventricle.
   D. inferior wall of the left ventricle.

6. It is decided that P.J. should receive reperfusion therapy. This is appropriate because
   A. acute ischemia is usually caused by a thrombus in the coronary artery.
   B. it reverses the atherosclerotic process in the coronary arteries.
   C. it decreases myocardial oxygen consumption.
   D. it relaxes smooth muscle and prevents coronary vasospasm.

7. At the time of admission, a blood sample is taken to determine whether P.J. has suffered an MI. Which of the following laboratory findings would indicate an MI?
   A. Elevated creatine phosphate
   B. Elevated total creatine kinase
   C. Elevated troponin I
   D. Elevated erythrocyte sedimentation rate

8. While P.J. is recovering from his cardiac event, he is monitored by continuous electrocardiography. On the day after hospital admission, he is noted to have a heart rate of 64 beats/min and a PR interval of 0.22 second. The QRS is normal, and there is one P wave for each QRS complex. This rhythm is termed
   A. sinus bradycardia.
   B. normal sinus rhythm.
   C. first-degree heart block.
   D. sinus arrhythmia.

9. P.J. is tolerating the rhythm well with no symptoms. Which of the following actions would be appropriate to take at this time?
   A. Prepare to insert a pacemaker.
   B. Administer atropine.
   C. Do nothing; this is a normal rhythm.
   D. Continue monitoring and assessing for symptoms.

10. Therapeutic interventions for P.J. are focused on increasing the oxygen supplied to the heart and decreasing the heart's demand for oxygen. Measures that reduce demand include using
    A. antiplatelet drugs.
    B. anticoagulants.
    C. morphine sulfate.
    D. thrombolytic drugs.

K.C. is an 86-year-old woman in generally good health who presents to the clinic with complaints of increasing shortness of breath and reduced activity tolerance. She has no significant cardiac history. Her blood pressure is 110/60 mm Hg, and her heart rate is 92 beats/min. There is a grade IV systolic murmur that radiates to the neck.

11. Considering K.C.'s age and the nature of the cardiac murmur, this is most likely
    A. mitral stenosis.
    B. mitral regurgitation.
    C. aortic stenosis.
    D. aortic regurgitation.

12. Auscultation of K.C.'s chest reveals bilateral fine crackles in the bases bilaterally, indicating
    A. right-sided heart failure.
    B. left-sided heart failure.
    C. pneumonia.
    D. acute respiratory distress syndrome.

13. K.C. is scheduled for surgical valve replacement and recovers well. Her ejection fraction after surgery is about 0.40. The ejection fraction is calculated
    A. the same as the stroke volume.
    B. as the stroke volume divided by the end-diastolic volume.
    C. as stroke volume divided by heart rate.
    D. as cardiac output divided by vascular resistance.

14. An ejection fraction of 0.40 indicates
    A. mild systolic dysfunction.
    B. mild diastolic dysfunction.
    C. moderate diastolic dysfunction.
    D. no significant left ventricular dysfunction.

15. K.C. is discharged on an ACE inhibitor medication. These drugs decrease mortality. What other group of drugs also accomplishes this?
    A. Digoxin
    B. Specific β-blockers
    C. Nitrates
    D. Diuretics

K.K. is a 20-year-old man who was completely healthy until he collapsed during a collegiate basketball game. He was resuscitated on the court and transported to the hospital.

16. Evaluation of K.K.'s 12-lead ECG reveals significant left ventricular hypertrophy but no evidence of ischemia. His heart rate is 60 beats/min, and his blood pressure is 116/70 mm Hg. Considering these findings and the above scenario, K.K. should be evaluated for
    A. coronary heart disease.
    B. hypertensive heart disease.
    C. hypertrophic cardiomyopathy.
    D. myocarditis.

17. K.K.'s echocardiogram demonstrates extreme septal hypertrophy, and so his collapse on the basketball court is attributed to
    A. an acute MI.
    B. an abnormal ventricular conduction pathway.
    C. an acute myocardial regurgitation.
    D. an acute aortic outflow obstruction.

18. The decision is made to perform a procedure to reduce the septum. Postoperatively, K.K.'s ECG demonstrates frequent nonconducted P waves (dropped beats) with a consistent PR interval for conducted beats and a wide QRS interval. This rhythm is called
    A. first-degree block.
    B. second-degree block, Mobitz type 1 (Wenckebach).
    C. second-degree block, Mobitz type 2.
    D. third-degree block.

19. Which of the following is the most appropriate response to K.K.'s rhythm disturbance?
    A. Monitor only; this rhythm rarely progresses.
    B. Prepare to initiate ventricular pacing if the block is symptomatic or progresses.
    C. Initiate antidysrhythmic medications.
    D. Administer atropine to increase the heart rate.

20. K.K.'s family should be advised that his disorder
    A. is genetic and family members should be evaluated.
    B. requires absolute activity restriction.
    C. is cured by surgery, and no further therapy is necessary.
    D. will progress to heart failure within a few years.

21 Respiratory Function and Alterations in Gas Exchange

MATCHING

1. Match each of the following anatomic terms with the appropriate letter in the figure.

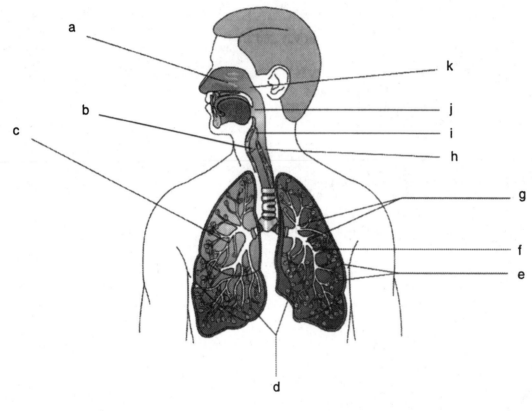

_____ Alveoli		_____ Nasopharynx	
_____ Nasal cavity		_____ Bronchioles	
_____ Bronchi		_____ Oropharynx	
_____ Esophagus		_____ Trachea	
_____ Right lung of patient		_____ Left lung of patient	
_____ Laryngopharynx			

TRUE/FALSE

Indicate whether the following statements regarding the anatomy and physiology of the respiratory system are true (T) or false (F).

2. _____ The larynx is anatomically part of the lower airway but performs functions characteristic of the upper airway.

3. _____ Cilia are located throughout the airway and are responsible for the production of mucus.

4. _____ Aspiration of food into the airway is prevented by closure of the trachea with swallowing.

5. _____ The carina is the anatomic end of the trachea, where the two mainstem bronchi originate.

6. _____ Aspirated materials tend to go into the right mainstem bronchus because it is shorter, wider, and at less of an angle from the trachea.

7. _____ The right lung has two lobes, whereas the left lung has three.

8. _____ Surfactant is produced by the columnar epithelial cells lining the airways.

9. _____ Stimulation of the sympathetic branch of the autonomic nervous system results in the release of acetylcholine, which causes constriction of smooth muscle in the bronchi and bronchioles.

10. _____ Cough reflex receptors are located at the epiglottis and carina.

11. _____ Gas exchange occurs between the alveoli and capillaries (alveolar unit) by the physical process of diffusion.

12. _____ A reduction in the number of alveoli commonly occurs as a part of the aging process.

13. _____ Blood is delivered to the lungs by the pulmonary vein, and oxygenated blood leaves the lungs via the pulmonary artery.

14. _____ Expiration normally is a passive process, primarily caused by the elastic recoil of the lung tissue.

15. _____ An increase in lung compliance is associated with aging.

16. _____ The chemoreceptors in the medulla are stimulated primarily by an increase in arterial CO_2.

MULTIPLE CHOICE

Select the one best answer to each of the following questions.

17. The zones of the lung are characterized by differences in
    A. alveolar ventilation.
    B. blood flow or perfusion.
    C. ventilation mismatch.
    D. partial pressure of oxygen.

18. A region of the lung that has poor ventilation and alveolar hypoxia has a
    A. low $\dot{V}/\dot{Q}$ ratio.
    B. high $\dot{V}/\dot{Q}$ ratio.
    C. elevated anatomic dead space.
    D. reduced airway resistance.

19. A patient with a low Pao_2 who does not improve with oxygen administration likely has a
    A. high $\dot{V}/\dot{Q}$ ratio.
    B. low $\dot{V}/\dot{Q}$ ratio.
    C. excessive dead space.
    D. intrapulmonary shunt (true shunt).

73

20. Administration of supplemental oxygen to a patient with poor alveolar ventilation will
    A. increase ventilation.
    B. reduce Pa_{CO_2}.
    C. reduce $\dot{V}/\dot{Q}$ imbalance.
    D. increase Pa_{O_2}.

21. Hyperventilation is diagnosed when a person has
    A. an elevated respiratory rate.
    B. an elevated Pa_{O_2}.
    C. a low Pa_{CO_2}.
    D. a high tidal volume.

FILL IN THE BLANKS

Fill in the blanks with the appropriate word or words.

22. Pulmonary hypertension is defined as a sustained increase in pulmonary artery systolic pressure above _____ mm Hg.

23. A significant increase in the resistance of the pulmonary vasculature results in pulmonary _____.

24. The three risk factors for thrombus formation, commonly called Virchow's triad, are

    1. _____,

    2. _____, and

    3. _____.

25. Lung cancers are rarely diagnosed before they _____, and therefore patients have a poor long-term survival rate.

26. The great majority of lung cancers occur in individuals who _____ _____.

27. A patient with a low $\dot{V}/\dot{Q}$ usually has a reduced arterial oxygen level. The severity of the $\dot{V}/\dot{Q}$ imbalance can be estimated by the difference in alveolar (Pa_{O_2}) and arterial (Pa_{O_2}) oxygen. Calculate the $A - aD_{O_2}$ for a patient at sea level (barometric pressure = 760 mm Hg) breathing room air (F_{IO_2} = 0.21) with a Pa_{O_2} of 60 mm Hg and a Pa_{CO_2} of 35 mm Hg. Use an R/Q value of 0.8 and a water vapor pressure of 47 mm Hg.

    The Pa_{O_2} is _____ mm Hg.

    The $A - aD_{O_2}$ is _____ mm Hg.

28. The patient in the previous question is given supplemental oxygen to achieve an F_{IO_2} of 0.40, and his blood gases are drawn again. The Pa_{O_2} is 100 mm Hg and the Pa_{CO_2} is 40 mm Hg. Calculate the $A - aD_{O_2}$ at this time, and determine if $\dot{V}/\dot{Q}$ has improved.

    The Pa_{O_2} is _____ mm Hg.

    The $A - aD_{O_2}$ is _____ mm Hg.

    Has $\dot{V}/\dot{Q}$ improved? _____ Explain your answer:

29. Diseases that cause global pulmonary hypoxemia usually are associated with pulmonary hypertension because hypoxemia causes _____ of pulmonary vessels.

30. An abnormal opening between the esophagus and the trachea is called a/an _____.

31. The conducting airways of the lung that are not involved in gas exchange are referred to as _____ _____.

32. Collapsed alveoli are the cause of the condition known as _____.

33. As the radius of the airway is reduced, as is the case with asthma attacks, the _____ to air flow increases.

34. Pulmonary compliance is a reflection of airway _____ and lung _____.

35. The respiratory centers of the brain are located in the _____ and _____.

22 Obstructive Pulmonary Disorders

1. *Compare and contrast chronic bronchitis and emphysema by filling in the table. Write "likely" or "unlikely" in the appropriate column.*

Characteristic	Chronic Bronchitis	Emphysema
Early hypoxemia		
Early CO_2 retention		
Productive cough		
Increased anteroposterior chest diameter		
Cor pulmonale		

MULTIPLE CHOICE

Select the one best answer to each of the following questions.

2. Bronchiolitis, commonly seen in infants due to respiratory syncytial virus, is characterized by
   A. airway inflammation and mucus formation.
   B. atrophy of smooth muscle of the airway.
   C. increased compliance of lung tissue.
   D. thin secretions from the nose.

3. Which of the following statements regarding cystic fibrosis is correct?
   A. It is caused by a bacterial infection.
   B. It can be prevented by a vaccine.
   C. It is associated with a genetic defect in chloride ion transport.
   D. It affects only the pulmonary system.

4. Signs or symptoms of tracheobronchial obstruction include all of the following *except*
   A. stridor.
   B. wheezing.
   C. sternal retractions.
   D. crackles.

5. A classic clinical finding when a patient has epiglottitis is
   A. pain and difficulty swallowing.
   B. pain with inspiration.
   C. unequal thoracic expansion.
   D. earaches.

6. Croup is a syndrome, a collection of signs and symptoms that may be caused by several etiologic factors. The most characteristic finding in croup is
   A. earaches.
   B. a barking cough with respiratory stridor.
   C. enlarged lymph nodes in the neck.
   D. marked fever.

76

7. Extrinsic/allergic asthma
   A. is mediated by IgG.
   B. presents with different signs and symptoms than intrinsic asthma.
   C. is caused by an antigen-antibody reaction on IgE-bearing mast cells.
   D. often is precipitated by exercise.

8. Air trapping associated with chronic obstructive diseases results in an increase in which of the following components of pulmonary function testing?
   A. Residual volume
   B. Forced expiratory volume in one second (FEV_1)
   C. Vital capacity
   D. Expiratory reserve volume

9. Acute and chronic bronchitis differ in which of the following ways?
   A. Chronic bronchitis is caused by repeated infections.
   B. Acute bronchitis is not associated with increased mucus production.
   C. Acute bronchitis produces arterial blood gas changes reflecting significant hypoxemia.
   D. Chronic bronchitis results in airway changes that are irreversible.

10. High-dose oxygen therapy must be used cautiously in patients with chronic bronchitis because
    A. $\dot{V}/\dot{Q}$ changes can result in further elevations in partial pressure of carbon dioxide in arterial blood ($Paco_2$).
    B. pulmonary vasoconstriction will worsen, increasing the work of the right side of the heart.
    C. respiratory smooth muscle constriction will result in increased air trapping.
    D. peripheral chemoreceptors will be depressed, and the patient will stop breathing.

11. Which of the following assessment findings is indicative of an asthma attack?
    A. Wheezing
    B. Thin, watery mucus production
    C. Runny nose
    D. Fever

12. Pathophysiologic differences between emphysema and chronic bronchitis include the fact that
    A. emphysema is characterized by hypersecretion of goblet and mucus cells.
    B. chronic bronchitis commonly results in polycythemia to compensate for persistent hypoxemia.
    C. chronic bronchitis destroys alveolar walls.
    D. emphysema is caused by chronic inflammation resulting in fibrotic airways.

13. Arterial blood gases for a patient with mild to moderate emphysema would reflect
    A. severe hypoxemia.
    B. increased $Paco_2$.
    C. near-normal Pao_2 and normal to low $Paco_2$.
    D. respiratory failure.

14. Pursed-lip breathing is commonly used by patients with emphysema because it
    A. increases the pressure gradient for gas exchange.
    B. helps strengthen accessory respiratory muscles.
    C. decreases small airway collapse during expiration.
    D. prolongs inspiration to allow gas to reach distal air sacs.

15. Clinical findings of prolonged hypoxemia in long-standing cystic fibrosis include
    A. cough.
    B. frequent respiratory infections.
    C. clubbing of the fingers.
    D. crackles in the lungs.

16. Decreased airway radius occurs in chronic bronchitis due to all of the following *except*
    A. increased elastic recoil.
    B. excessive amounts of sputum.
    C. airway scarring.
    D. inflammation.

TRUE/FALSE

Indicate whether each of the following statements is true (T) or false (F).

17. _____ Emphysema is associated with chronic neutrophil production of elastase in the lung.

18. _____ A patient who has a significant increase in FEV_1 in response to bronchodilator therapy would be diagnosed with chronic obstructive pulmonary disease (COPD).

19. _____ Bronchodilator therapy with a β-receptor agonist, such as albuterol, treats the underlying cause of asthma (inflammation).

20. _____ The majority of patients who are diagnosed with COPD have both chronic bronchitis and emphysematous changes.

21. _____ An elevated total lung capacity, residual volume, and functional residual capacity are characteristic of obstructive lung disorders.

FILL IN THE BLANKS

Fill in the blanks with the appropriate word or words.

22. Regardless of the trigger for an asthma attack, all forms are characterized by airway _____, which causes mucosal edema, bronchoconstriction, and hypersecretion of mucus.

23. The increased work of breathing during an asthma attack is attributed to increased airway _____.

24. The peak expiratory flow rate is characteristically _____ in obstructive lung disorders but normal or _____ in restrictive disorders.

25. A patient with a significant smoking history, chronically elevated Pa_{CO_2}, and hypoxemia most likely has a respiratory disease diagnosis of _____ _____.

26. Emphysema is a chronic obstructive lung disorder associated with loss of lung parenchymal tissue. Obstruction occurs because lung parenchyma is responsible for maintaining _____ _____ on the small airways.

27. A low, flat diaphragm; narrow mediastinum; and decreased lung density on chest x-ray are characteristic findings in _____.

28. Interventions for the patient with asthma are often based on the assessment of _____ _____.

29. Acute airway obstruction with a foreign object may be relieved by _____ _____ or the _____ _____.

30. During pulmonary function testing, bronchospasm may be pharmacologically induced. This is known as _____ _____.

23 Restrictive Pulmonary Disorders

TRUE/FALSE

Indicate whether each of the following statements is true (T) or false (F).

1. _____ A patient with a positive PPD tuberculin test might not have active tuberculosis.

2. _____ Surfactant is a phospholipid mixture that reduces alveolar surface tension.

3. _____ Pneumothorax is characterized by a finding of increased density (white out) on x-ray.

4. _____ Fibrotic lung disorders are characterized by reduced lung compliance and decreased tidal volumes.

5. _____ Patients with significant fibrotic lung changes tend to breathe more slowly to allow more time in the exhalation phase.

MULTIPLE CHOICE

Select the one best answer to each of the following questions.

6. Restrictive pulmonary disorders are associated with which of the following pulmonary function test results?
   A. Increased total lung capacity
   B. Increased residual volume
   C. Decreased peak flow rate
   D. Decreased vital capacity

7. Occupational lung diseases such as pneumoconiosis
   A. result from chronic inhalation of inert dust particles.
   B. are characterized by early marked elevations in Pa_{CO_2}.
   C. produce an increase in lung compliance.
   D. are caused by antigen-antibody reactions.

8. The pathology of acute respiratory distress syndrome produces hypoxemia that is refractory to oxygen therapy. This is because of
   A. decreased pulmonary compliance.
   B. increased functional residual capacity.
   C. intrapulmonary shunt (true shunt).
   D. significant dyspnea.

9. The underlying pathologic condition of infant respiratory distress syndrome (hyaline membrane disease) is primarily
   A. increased numbers of red blood cells slowing perfusion.
   B. deficiency of surfactant increasing alveolar surface tension and causing atelectasis.
   C. right-to-left shunting of blood through a patent ductus arteriosus.
   D. epithelial cell damage causing edema.

10. A tension pneumothorax would present with
    A. tracheal deviation and mediastinal shift away from the pneumothorax.
    B. minimal effect on the blood pressure or pulse.
    C. flattened neck veins due to decreased venous return to the heart.
    D. hyperresonance to percussion and bronchial breath sounds over the uninvolved lung.

11. A pleural effusion may develop when a patient with liver disease is unable to synthesize adequate amounts of albumin. This would result in fluid movement from the vascular bed to the pleural space because of
    A. increased pleural capillary hydrostatic pressure.
    B. increased pleural interstitial pressure.
    C. decreased pleural capillary oncotic pressure.
    D. decreased intrapleural pressure.

12. The primary feature distinguishing bacterial from viral pneumonia is
    A. a cough productive of purulent sputum.
    B. decreased breath sounds.
    C. atelectasis.
    D. tachycardia.

13. Transmission of *Mycobacterium tuberculosis* is primarily via
    A. contaminated blood.
    B. inhaled droplets.
    C. sexual intercourse.
    D. contaminated skin that has been in contact with contaminated articles.

14. Those who survive acute respiratory distress syndrome commonly have
    A. no chronic lung changes.
    B. an increased risk for lung cancer.
    C. chronic restrictive lung changes.
    D. right-sided heart failure.

15. Risk of secondary pneumothorax is increased in patients who
    A. are tall, thin, and male.
    B. have emphysema.
    C. have thoracic trauma.
    D. are allergic.

16. Amyotrophic lateral sclerosis
    A. only involves the diaphragm and intercostal muscles.
    B. is transitory and recovery is complete.
    C. leads to death by respiratory failure.
    D. is caused by damage at the myoneural junction.

17. Risk of aspiration pneumonia is especially increased in patients with
    A. a decreased level of consciousness.
    B. increased age.
    C. chronic respiratory disease.
    D. viral pneumonia.

FILL IN THE BLANKS

Fill in the blanks with the appropriate word or words.

18. Pleural effusions low in protein such as those caused by liver failure are called _____, whereas those high in protein such as those due to lung cancer are called _____.

19. Hypoventilation associated with obesity is caused by _____ work of breathing.

20. When a patient has a flail chest, the free segment moves inward on _____ and outward on _____.

21. The classic chest x-ray finding associated with pulmonary tuberculosis is a calcified nodule with a necrotic center called a _____ _____.

22. _____ pneumonia produces an exudate, whereas _____ pneumonia does not.

23. The acid-base abnormality most often seen with early restrictive lung diseases is _____ _____.

24. The majority of cases of scoliosis are diagnosed in the _____ age group.

25. Bacterial pneumonia may produce a pulmonary effusion composed of infected material; this is called a/an _____.

26. Tuberculosis is spread by _____ _____.

27. Severe acute respiratory syndrome (SARS) is caused by a _____.

28. Although many factors can trigger the development of fibrotic interstitial lung diseases, they share a common pathogenesis of interstitial _____ and immune-mediated injury.

29. The fibrotic lung disease called anthracosis is a result of inhalation of _____ _____.

30. Positive end-expiratory pressure (PEEP) therapy is used in patients with acute respiratory distress syndrome (ARDS) to increase _____ _____ capacity.

UNIT VI: Case Studies

J.B. is a 46-year-old asthmatic woman who has been hospitalized with a bacterial pneumonia primarily involving the right middle and lower lobes. Antibiotics and oxygen therapy at F_{IO_2} 0.28 by nasal cannula are initiated. A pulse oximeter is ordered to monitor oxygen saturation.

1. J.B.'s oxygen saturation is likely to be lowest when she is positioned
   A. in a high Fowler position.
   B. lying on her left side.
   C. lying on her right side.
   D. lying supine with the head of the bed flat.

2. Using the "law of 5s," J.B.'s ideal P_{AO_2} level is estimated to be
   A. 84 mm Hg.
   B. 280 mm Hg.
   C. 140 mm Hg.
   D. 28 mm Hg.

3. The combined pathophysiologic conditions of asthma and bacterial pneumonia increase the risk for J.B. to develop
   A. hypoxemia.
   B. weakened respiratory muscles.
   C. apnea.
   D. increased residual volume.

4. Common manifestations of bacterial pneumonia include all of the following *except*
   A. fever.
   B. productive cough.
   C. tachypnea.
   D. hyperinflation.

5. J.B.'s fever can be expected to alter her oxyhemoglobin saturation curve by
   A. shifting it to the right.
   B. shifting it to the left.
   C. inducing no change.
   D. increasing the affinity of hemoglobin for oxygen.

6. Asthma is an obstructive disease, whereas pneumonia is a restrictive one. A major difference between restrictive and obstructive pulmonary diseases is that in restrictive diseases
   A. lung tissue itself is not involved in the disease process.
   B. peak expiratory flow is not decreased.
   C. lung compliance is not altered.
   D. the inflammatory process is not part of the pathologic condition.

M.R. is a 63-year-old man who has had emphysema for many years. The nurse is on a home visit, meeting M.R. for the first time.

7. In performing a physical assessment, the nurse notes the patient has a "barrel" configuration to the chest. This is a consequence of
   A. reduced intrapleural pressures.
   B. bronchial airway expansion.
   C. increased vital capacity.
   D. increased residual lung volume.

8. A common symptom in patients with emphysema is
   A. nausea.
   B. significant sputum production.
   C. dyspnea.
   D. pleuritic chest pain.

9. M.R. and other patients with emphysema are at risk for which of the following complications because of the pathophysiologic process of their disease?
   A. Cancer
   B. Pneumothorax
   C. Pleural effusion
   D. Tuberculosis

10. M.R., like most patients with emphysema, is able to maintain relatively normal arterial blood gases until the disease is very advanced. This is primarily because of
   A. secondary polycythemia.
   B. increased tidal volumes.
   C. increased respiratory effort.
   D. a slowly enlarging right side of the heart.

11. M.R., with his chronic obstructive pulmonary disease, exerts most of his work of breathing during the _____ phase of respiration, whereas patients with restrictive diseases exert most of their work of breathing during the _____ phase.

12. With advanced emphysema, M.R. has a large alveolar-arterial oxygen difference $(A - aDo_2)$, which means he
   A. always has significant hypoxemia.
   B. is hypoventilating.
   C. has an enlarged zone 2 of the lung.
   D. has poor lung function and impaired gas exchange.

Five-year-old P.T. is brought to the clinic for a routine evaluation of his cystic fibrosis.

13. The underlying pathologic process of cystic fibrosis is related to
    A. excessively thick mucus production in the lungs.
    B. decreased mucus degeneration by enzyme systems.
    C. primary surfactant deficiency.
    D. pulmonary vascular destruction.

14. Patients with cystic fibrosis are likely to develop
    A. venous thrombi.
    B. respiratory infections.
    C. diabetes mellitus.
    D. dysrhythmias.

15. Therapeutic interventions for cystic fibrosis include all of the following *except*
    A. postural drainage.
    B. nutritional supplementation.
    C. prophylactic antibiotic coverage.
    D. chloride ion supplementation.

H.J. has been hospitalized following an automobile accident. Several ribs were broken, resulting in a pneumothorax. He is being treated with a closed-chest drainage system and oxygen by nasal cannula titrated to keep his Sao$_2$ at 90% or higher.

16. Pneumothorax is
    A. a collection of pus in the pleural space.
    B. a collection of air in the pleural space.
    C. a collection of air in the alveolar blebs.
    D. a puncture in the chest wall.

17. Typical presentation of a pneumothorax includes
    A. an elevated white blood cell count.
    B. elevated blood pressure.
    C. decreased lung sounds on the affected side.
    D. increased lung sounds on the unaffected side.

18. Closed-chest drainage systems work to reexpand a lung after pneumothorax by
    A. reestablishing the normal negative intrapleural pressure.
    B. creating a positive pressure in the pleural space.
    C. removing excess fluid from the pleural space so that there is room for lung expansion.
    D. pulling oxygen into distal air sacs to reexpand lung tissue.

Three-year-old R.C. is brought to the emergency department by her parents. They report that she seems to be having a great deal of difficulty getting a breath and has a coarse, barking cough. The nurse practitioner diagnoses croup.

19. Parents of children with croup typically report that the child has recently had
    A. routine immunizations.
    B. an upper respiratory infection.
    C. a high fever.
    D. no recent change in health or activity.

20. Differentiation of croup from epiglottitis is essential because
    A. the two diseases require different antibiotic therapies.
    B. croup is usually viral in origin.
    C. humidified treatments for croup will worsen epiglottitis.
    D. epiglottitis can cause rapid and complete airway obstruction.

21. Assessment findings in a child with croup include
    A. digital clubbing.
    B. a prolonged expiratory phase.
    C. expiratory wheezing.
    D. retractions of intercostal muscles with inspiration.

24 Fluid and Electrolyte Homeostasis and Imbalances

TRUE/FALSE

Indicate whether each of the following statements regarding fluid–electrolyte balance is true (T) or false (F).

1. _____ The principal regulators of fluid intake are thirst and habit.

2. _____ Fluid movement across the capillary wall is determined by filtration pressure.

3. _____ Electrolyte movement across the capillary wall is determined by diffusion.

4. _____ The principal determinant of capillary filtration is interstitial hydrostatic pressure.

5. _____ Osmosis is an active, energy-requiring process.

6. _____ Water moves across cell membranes according to osmotic gradients.

7. _____ Two thirds of the total body fluid is contained in the extracellular space.

8. _____ When isotonic fluids are administered, they remain in the extracellular space and do not enter the cells.

9. _____ When water is administered, it distributes among all fluid compartments by osmosis.

10. _____ Aldosterone is a hormone that promotes reabsorption of free water in the collecting tubule.

11. _____ Antidiuretic hormone (ADH) induces the kidney to produce concentrated urine.

12. _____ The concentrations of potassium, magnesium, phosphate, and calcium are all higher in the extracellular fluid compartment than within the cell.

COMPLETION

Evaluate the following laboratory values and write (N) for normal, (H) for abnormally high, or (L) for abnormally low.

13. _____ Serum potassium: 3.8 mEq/L

14. _____ Serum calcium: 9.5 mg/dL

15. _____ Serum sodium: 149 mEq/L

16. _____ Serum Mg^{2+}: 6.0 mEq/L

17. _____ Serum P_i: 2.0 mEq/L

COMPARE/CONTRAST

Compare and contrast electrolyte disorders by filling in the following tables.

18.

Characteristic	Hypernatremia	Hyponatremia
Etiologic factor		
Clinical findings		
Treatment		

19.

Characteristic	Hyperkalemia	Hypokalemia
Etiologic factor		
Clinical findings		
Treatment		

20.

Characteristic	Hypercalcemia	Hypocalcemia
Etiologic factor		
Clinical findings		
Treatment		

21.

Characteristic	Hypermagnesemia	Hypomagnesemia
Etiologic factor		
Clinical findings		
Treatment		

22.

Characteristic	Hyperphosphatemia	Hypophosphatemia
Etiologic factor		
Clinical findings		
Treatment		

Select the one best answer to each of the following questions.

23. Saline deficit is defined as
    A. a deficit of extracellular volume.
    B. a deficit of serum sodium.
    C. a deficit of body water.
    D. hyponatremia.

24. Signs and symptoms of saline deficit include
    A. low serum sodium.
    B. increased serum osmolality.
    C. postural hypotension.
    D. seizures.

25. Water excess (hyponatremia) is best detected by
    A. weight changes.
    B. blood pressure changes.
    C. low serum sodium.
    D. edema.

26. Conditions that predispose to hyponatremia include
    A. high rates of isotonic fluid administration.
    B. significant blood loss.
    C. insufficient production of ADH.
    D. excessive administration of 5% dextrose in water (D_5W).

27. If a patient with a normal serum sodium is given 1 L of normal saline, how much of that volume will distribute into the intracellular space?
    A. None
    B. One third
    C. Two thirds
    D. All

28. If a patient is given 1 L of D_5W, how much of that volume will distribute to the intracellular space?
    A. None
    B. One third
    C. Two thirds
    D. All

29. The most appropriate fluid for treating a patient with a normal serum sodium and an extracellular volume deficit is
    A. whole blood.
    B. isotonic fluid (e.g., normal saline).
    C. D_5W.
    D. unrestricted oral water.

30. Generalized edema is usually a consequence of
    A. excessive extracellular volume.
    B. reduced plasma proteins.
    C. high blood pressure.
    D. increased capillary hydrostatic pressure.

31. Dependent edema is usually a consequence of
    A. hyponatremia.
    B. reduced plasma proteins.
    C. high arterial blood pressure.
    D. increased capillary hydrostatic pressure.

32. The plasma concentration of an electrolyte correlates most closely with
    A. the intracellular concentration.
    B. the interstitial concentration.
    C. the urinary concentration.
    D. the cerebrospinal fluid concentration.

33. Muscle weakness may be a symptom of all of the following electrolyte disturbances *except*
    A. hyperkalemia.
    B. hypercalcemia.
    C. hypermagnesemia.
    D. hyperphosphatemia.

34. Manifestations of potassium imbalance are attributed to
    A. an altered threshold for excitation.
    B. an altered resting membrane potential.
    C. an altered release of neurotransmitter at the neuromuscular junction.
    D. an altered production of intracellular adenosine triphosphate (ATP).

35. Manifestations of magnesium imbalance are attributed to
    A. an altered threshold for excitation.
    B. an altered resting membrane potential.
    C. an altered release of neurotransmitter at the neuromuscular junction.
    D. an altered production of intracellular ATP.

36. Manifestations of calcium imbalance are attributed to
    A. an altered threshold for excitation.
    B. an altered resting membrane potential.
    C. altered release of neurotransmitter at the neuromuscular junction.
    D. altered production of intracellular ATP.

37. Fluid volume excess may be due to all of the following *except*
    A. excessive isotonic fluid administration.
    B. adrenal gland failure.
    C. heart failure.
    D. renal failure.

FILL IN THE BLANKS

Fill in the blanks with the appropriate word or words.

38. A patient exhibiting edema, weight gain, and a normal serum sodium level probably has a fluid imbalance called

    _____ _____.

39. Hypernatremia and increased serum osmolality are associated with a deficit of _____.

40. A normal serum potassium level is between _____ and _____ mEq/L.

41. A high serum potassium level causes the resting membrane potential to be _____, whereas a low serum

    potassium level causes _____ resting membrane potential.

42. While having his blood pressure taken with a cuff inflated around the upper arm, a patient complains of tingling and

    spasms of the hand. These symptoms are called a positive _____ sign and usually are a consequence of

    _____ or _____.

43. A patient who presents with unexplained hypercalcemia should be evaluated for _____ as the cause.

44. When a pregnant woman with preeclampsia is given a magnesium infusion to suppress seizures during delivery, one should anticipate that the newborn may exhibit neuromuscular and respiratory _____.

45. Normally the relationship of serum calcium and serum phosphate is _____; this means that when calcium is elevated, phosphate is _____, and when calcium is low, phosphate is _____.

25 Acid–Base Homeostasis and Imbalances

TRUE/FALSE

Indicate whether each of the following statements regarding the anatomy and physiology of acid–base balance is true (T) or false (F).

1. _____ The normal ratio of bicarbonate to carbonic acid is 10:1.

2. _____ A pH buffer releases H^+ when the pH is high and binds H^+ when the pH is low.

3. _____ The bicarbonate buffer system is the most important pH buffer in the extracellular fluid.

4. _____ The kidneys control the level of bicarbonate in the extracellular fluid.

5. _____ An acid accepts hydrogen ions.

6. _____ The pH measured in the blood is always the same as that within cerebrospinal fluid and cells.

7. _____ When the pH is lower than the normal serum range, it is called acidic.

8. _____ H^+ in the urine can be buffered to form ammonium ions.

COMPLETION

Evaluate the following laboratory values and write (N) for normal, (H) for abnormally high, or (L) for abnormally low.

9. _____ $Paco_2$: 30 mm Hg

10. _____ Arterial pH: 7.38

11. _____ Arterial HCO_3-: 24 mEq/L

Analyze the following arterial blood gas results, identifying the abnormality and whether it is metabolic or respiratory in origin, and then whether there are appropriate changes in the direction of compensation (Yes or No).

12. pH = 7.46; $Paco_2$ = 30; HCO_3- = 19

Abnormality _____ Origin _____ Compensation _____

13. pH = 7.30; $Paco_2$ = 51; HCO_3- = 23

Abnormality _____ Origin _____ Compensation _____

14. pH = 7.36; $Paco_2$ = 29; HCO_3- = 20

Abnormality _____ Origin _____ Compensation _____

MULTIPLE CHOICE

Select the one best answer to each of the following questions.

15. The role of the lungs in maintaining acid–base balance includes
    A. elimination of metabolic acids.
    B. elimination of excess H^+.
    C. production of bicarbonate.
    D. elimination of carbonic acids.

16. In response to a chronically elevated $Paco_2$, the kidneys would be expected to compensate by
    A. excreting more bicarbonate.
    B. producing more bicarbonate.
    C. reabsorbing more hydrogen ions.
    D. filtering more bicarbonate.

17. Which of the following arterial blood gases would be categorized as compensated metabolic acidosis?
    A. pH 7.39, $Paco_2$ 32, HCO_3^- 18
    B. pH 7.31, $Paco_2$ 37, HCO_3^- 18
    C. pH 7.45, $Paco_2$ 32, HCO_3^- 23
    D. pH 7.40, $Paco_2$ 39, HCO_3^- 24

18. A blood gas with pH 7.24, $Paco_2$ 58, and HCO_3^- 24 would be categorized as
    A. metabolic acidosis.
    B. metabolic alkalosis.
    C. respiratory acidosis.
    D. respiratory alkalosis.

19. Metabolic acidosis is associated with all of the following *except*
    A. diarrhea.
    B. vomiting.
    C. end-stage kidney disease.
    D. ketoacidosis.

20. Which of the following statements regarding respiratory acidosis is *true*?
    A. It can occur in a prolonged, severe asthma attack.
    B. The pH is elevated.
    C. A decreased respiratory rate would be compensatory.
    D. There is an increase in neuron excitability in motor neurons.

FILL IN THE BLANKS

Fill in the blanks with the appropriate word or words.

21. A normal blood pH can be maintained despite variances in HCO_3^- and carbonic acid as long as their ratio is maintained at _____.

22. The amount of H^+ excreted in the urine can be increased by combining the H^+ with urine buffers in the following reactions: _____; _____.

23. In general, acidosis produces central nervous system _____, and alkalosis produces central nervous system _____.

24. When two primary imbalances develop simultaneously due to two different pathologies, it is called a _____ _____ _____.

25. When the mother of a child in the emergency room hyperventilates due to anxiety, she may develop a _____ _____.

Joe is a 24-year-old man brought to the emergency department by a friend. The friend reports that Joe spent the day on the lake in a boat and then developed severe headache and vomiting in the evening. He has been unable to keep down any fluids, and he is warm and flushed, with a temperature of 102° F. He has not urinated in the last 16 hours.

1. Joe's blood pressure is 90/50 mm Hg, and his heart rate is 118 beats/min when he is supine. When at the nurse's request he attempts to sit up for an orthostatic blood pressure reading, he becomes faint and must lie down. These findings are consistent with a diagnosis of
   A. saline deficit.
   B. hyponatremia.
   C. renal failure.
   D. cardiogenic shock.

2. Laboratory analysis of Joe's blood reveals that his serum sodium is 150 mEq/L, indicating
   A. saline excess.
   B. water deficit.
   C. hyponatremia.
   D. a normal value.

3. An intravenous line is established to provide fluid replacement. The most appropriate fluid for expanding Joe's extracellular volume to improve his blood pressure and heart rate is
   A. water.
   B. 5% dextrose in water.
   C. normal saline (0.9%).
   D. half-normal saline (0.045%).

4. Joe received 3 L of isotonic fluid, and his blood pressure stabilized at 110/70 mm Hg with a heart rate of 80 beats/min while he was supine. When Joe stood up, his blood pressure dropped to 100/60 mm Hg with a heart rate of 96 beats/min. This indicates that
   A. Joe has received adequate fluid replacement therapy.
   B. Joe's intravenous fluid should be changed to a hypotonic fluid.
   C. Joe needs more isotonic fluid replacement.
   D. Joe is not responding to fluid therapy.

5. For which acid–base disorder is Joe at risk if his vomiting continues for a prolonged period?
   A. Respiratory acidosis
   B. Respiratory alkalosis
   C. Metabolic acidosis
   D. Metabolic alkalosis

Cindy is a 16-year-old girl with type 1 (insulin-dependent) diabetes. In addition to her morning and evening doses of insulin, she is to monitor her blood glucose four times daily and supplement the insulin as needed. For the past several weeks, Cindy has been extremely busy with school activities and has not been monitoring her blood glucose carefully. She is now in the clinic complaining of severe fatigue and abdominal pain.

6. A urine sample reveals the presence of ketones. What acid–base disorder may accompany excessive ketone production?
   A. Respiratory acidosis
   B. Respiratory alkalosis
   C. Metabolic acidosis
   D. Metabolic alkalosis

7. An arterial blood gas sample is obtained, which shows a pH of 7.38, $Paco_2$ of 33, and HCO_3^- of 19 mEq/L. This blood gas result is consistent with a diagnosis of
   A. metabolic acidosis.
   B. metabolic alkalosis.
   C. respiratory alkalosis.
   D. respiratory alkalosis.

8. What action would be most appropriate at this time to manage this acid–base disorder?
   A. Manage the underlying problem with insulin.
   B. Administer sodium bicarbonate to normalize the HCO_3^-.
   C. Have the patient breathe into a paper bag to normalize the $Paco_2$.
   D. Do nothing; this is a normal blood gas result.

9. An electrolyte disorder that often accompanies diabetic ketosis is
   A. hyponatremia.
   B. hypochloremia.
   C. hyperkalemia.
   D. hypophosphatemia.

10. A finger-stick blood glucose sample shows a value of 336 mg/dL, and there is significant glycosuria. These two findings suggest that Cindy likely has a deficit of
   A. sodium bicarbonate.
   B. potassium.
   C. urine output.
   D. fluid volume.

George is a 64-year-old male with chronic bronchitis/chronic obstructive pulmonary disease (COPD). He has felt more short of breath and has had a fever for 2 days. When he arrives at the emergency department, he is noted to have a respiratory rate of 20 breaths/min and is feeling very dyspneic. He is using oxygen at 2 L per nasal cannula. A blood gas sample is obtained, with the following results: pH: 7.30: $Paco_2$: 62 mm Hg; HCO_3^-: 30 mEq/L; Pao_2: 60 mm Hg.

11. What is George's acid–base status?
   A. Respiratory acidosis
   B. Respiratory acidosis
   C. Metabolic alkalosis
   D. Mixed acidosis

12. The most appropriate therapy to improve George's acid–base imbalance is
   A. oxygen administration.
   B. measures to improve ventilation.
   C. sodium bicarbonate administration.
   D. reduction of his oxygen supplementation.

13. George is started on bronchodilator therapy and antibiotics and begins to improve. A repeat arterial blood gas is obtained, with the following results: pH: 7.37; $Paco_2$: 53 mm Hg; HCO_3^-: 30 mEq/L; Pao_2: 65 mm Hg. What is the most appropriate interpretation?
   A. Normal acid–base status
   B. Compensated respiratory alkalosis
   C. Compensated respiratory acidosis
   D. Compensated metabolic alkalosis

14. The improvement in George's acid–base status (compared to ABG from case scenario) can be attributed to
   A. increased alveolar ventilation.
   B. increased alveolar oxygenation.
   C. increased production of HCO_3^-.
   D. reduced dead space.

26 Renal Function

MATCHING

1. Match each of the following anatomic terms with the appropriate letter in the figure.

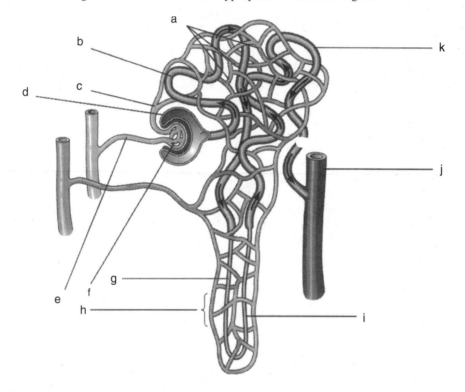

_____	Afferent arteriole	_____	Glomerulus
_____	Efferent arteriole	_____	Bowman capsule
_____	Ascending loop of Henle	_____	Peritubular capillaries
_____	Collecting tubule	_____	Vasa recta
_____	Proximal convoluted tubule	_____	Distal convoluted tubule
_____	Descending loop of Henle		

Match each definition on the left with its term on the right. Not all terms are defined.

2. _____ Functional unit of the kidney

3. _____ Percentage of the cardiac output delivered to the kidneys

4. _____ External landmark for the location of the kidneys

5. _____ Area of the kidney where the glomeruli and nephron tubules are located

6. _____ Area of the kidney receiving the smallest amount of blood

7. _____ Branch of the autonomic nervous system that controls intrarenal perfusion and the release of renin

8. _____ Movement of fluid from an area of higher pressure to an area of lower pressure; occurs in the glomerulus

9. _____ Area of the kidney where two thirds of the water and electrolytes are reabsorbed into the blood

10. _____ Area of the kidney where aldosterone acts to produce sodium and water reabsorption

11. _____ Area of the kidney where water is reabsorbed under the influence of antidiuretic hormone

12. _____ Loss of large molecules such as protein and blood cells is prevented by this

13. _____ Renal participation in acid–base balance is primarily through secretion of _____ and reabsorption and generation of _____

14. _____ Potassium balance is primarily controlled by the action of this hormone

15. _____ This hormone inhibits the effects of aldosterone, resulting in sodium and water elimination from the body

16. _____ Hypoxia causes the release of this hormone from the kidney

17. _____ Renal activation of this will allow absorption of dietary calcium

18. _____ Laboratory test that best reflects the glomerular filtration rate (GFR)

19. _____ Laboratory test affected by the hydration status and metabolic rate of the patient

20. _____ Active process in the tubules of moving potassium into the filtrate

A. Atrial natriuretic peptide
B. 50%
C. Basement membrane
D. Secretion
E. Medulla
F. Vitamin D
G. Aldosterone
H. Nephron
I. 20% to 25%
J. Serum creatinine
K. Parasympathetic nervous system
L. Proximal convoluted tubule
M. HPO_4^{2-}; NH_3
N. Erythropoietin
O. Costovertebral angle
P. Distal convoluted tubule
Q. H^+; HCO_3^-
R. BUN
S. Sympathetic nervous system
T. Retroperitoneal
U. Filtration
V. Excretion
W. Collecting ducts
X. Cortex
Y. Renal pelvis
Z. Renal biopsy

TRUE/FALSE

Indicate whether each of the following statements about renal function is true (T) or false (F).

21. _____ The thick ascending loop of Henle is impermeable to water.

22. _____ Water is actively transported across the renal tubules.

23. _____ The normal GFR in a healthy adult is about 60 mL/min.

24. _____ Constriction of the efferent arteriole of the glomerulus increases the GFR.

25. _____ Administration of angiotensin-converting enzyme inhibitors (ACEI) agents decreases the glomerular filtration pressure.

95

Fill in the blanks with the appropriate word or words.

26. A normal urinalysis may contain up to _____ red blood cells or white blood cells per high-powered field.

27. The presence of urinary casts is helpful in diagnosing certain kidney diseases: _____ casts signify pyelonephritis; _____ casts signify glomerulonephritis; and _____ _____ casts signify tubular necrosis and sloughing of tubule cells.

28. The noninvasive and painless diagnostic test that employs high-frequency sound waves to provide images of the kidneys and other components of the urinary system is called _____.

29. A diagnostic test used to determine the GFR in an individual is _____ _____ _____.

30. In the glomerulus, materials are filtered from the capillaries through _____ and between glomerular podocytes through _____ _____.

27 Intrarenal Disorders

Indicate whether the following statements are true (T) or false (F).

1. _____ The most common inherited congenital renal disorder is renal agenesis.

2. _____ An individual who develops nephrolithiasis has a better than 30% chance of experiencing another episode.

3. _____ The majority of tumors affecting the kidney are malignant.

4. _____ Nephrotic syndrome is a result of any condition that causes large amounts of protein to pass into the filtrate at the glomerular basement membrane.

5. _____ Only 10% of the cases of end-stage renal disease are due to glomerulopathies.

6. _____ Postinfectious causes are the most common causes of acute glomerulonephritis in children.

7. _____ The cause of acute urinary tract infections in both men and women is usually viral.

8. _____ The most common cause of chronic proteinuria is diabetes mellitus.

9. _____ Removal of indwelling catheters as soon as possible is an important preventive measure for acute pyelonephritis.

10. _____ Obstruction of the urinary tract results in stasis of urine flow and increased infection risk.

MULTIPLE CHOICE

Select the one best answer to each of the following questions.

11. Adult polycystic kidney disease
    A. is usually symptomatic by early adolescence.
    B. manifests with decreasing renal function and hypertension in adulthood.
    C. is seen as small, atrophied kidneys on ultrasound.
    D. is very responsive to treatment and ultimately curable.

12. Pain in the kidney, as occurs with pyelonephritis or trauma, is a result of
    A. the presence of abundant nociceptors throughout the kidney tissue.
    B. irritation of densely packed pain receptors in the renal pelvis.
    C. activation of afferent nerves of the corticospinal tracts.
    D. stimulation of nociceptors located in the renal capsule.

13. Acute glomerulonephritis
    A. relentlessly progresses to chronic renal failure.
    B. presents with the classic manifestations of fluid volume deficit and increased plasma oncotic pressure.
    C. is usually a result of reactions to antigen–antibody complexes in the glomerulus.
    D. produces a pathologic increase in the glomerular filtration rate (GFR).

14. Manifestations of nephrotic syndrome include all of the following *except*
    A. bleeding.
    B. edema.
    C. hyperlipidemia.
    D. hypoalbuminemia.

15. In chronic glomerulonephritis
    A. the cause is an overwhelming infection.
    B. progression to end-stage renal disease is common.
    C. complete remission of the disease is common.
    D. nephrons hypertrophy and the kidneys enlarge.

16. Nephroblastoma, or Wilms tumor, is the most common renal malignancy in children. Its diagnosis is
    A. followed by aggressive chemotherapy as the primary intervention.
    B. made on the basis of an abnormal urinalysis result.
    C. often suggested by a palpable mass in the flank or abdomen.
    D. grave because the prognosis is very poor in all cases.

17. The most common type of renal calculi (nephrolithiasis) is
    A. calcium oxalate.
    B. uric acid.
    C. cystine.
    D. struvite.

18. Movement of renal calculi into the ureter produces
    A. infection.
    B. a reduction in pain.
    C. bladder outflow obstruction.
    D. renal colic.

19. Risk factors for acute pyelonephritis include all of the following *except*
    A. diabetes mellitus.
    B. kidney trauma.
    C. vesicoureteral reflux.
    D. elderly age.

20. Renal cell carcinoma
    A. is a single histologic entity.
    B. usually originates in the medulla.
    C. risk is associated with a sedentary lifestyle.
    D. is usually asymptomatic until advanced stages.

21. The finding of white blood cell casts in the urine is indicative of
    A. cystitis.
    B. pyelonephritis.
    C. glomerulonephritis.
    D. acute tubular necrosis.

22. The finding of red blood cell casts in the urine is indicative of
    A. cystitis.
    B. pyelonephritis.
    C. glomerulonephritis.
    D. acute tubular necrosis.

23. The finding of chronic painless hematuria should be investigated because it may indicate
    A. nephrotic syndrome.
    B. renal cancer.
    C. urinary tract infection.
    D. chronic kidney disease.

24. The finding of renal tubular cell casts in the urine indicates
    A. nephrotic syndrome.
    B. glomerulonephritis.
    C. urinary tract infection.
    D. tubular necrosis.

25. Polycystic kidney disease is
    A. a genetic disorder.
    B. unlikely to progress to renal failure.
    C. reversible with appropriate therapy.
    D. a consequence of type 1 diabetes mellitus.

FILL IN THE BLANKS

Fill in the blanks with the appropriate word or words.

26. Renal calculi that develop following a urinary tract infection are composed of _____.

27. A child presenting with periorbital edema and hematuria should be evaluated for _____.

28. Plasmapheresis may be used to manage certain types of glomerulonephritis in which renal damage is caused by

    _____.

29. Diabetic nephropathy should be suspected in diabetic patients who have _____ in their urine.

30. The diagnostic test used to differentiate kidney tumors from cysts is _____.

28 Acute Kidney Injury and Chronic Kidney Disease

TRUE/FALSE

Indicate whether the following statements are true (T) or false (F).

1. _____ A tumor in the bladder could produce postrenal acute renal failure.

2. _____ One risk factor for the development of chronic kidney disease is simply aging.

3. _____ A common finding in the urinalysis of a patient with acute tubular necrosis (ATN) is increased protein and red blood cells.

4. _____ Elevated blood urea nitrogen (BUN) values seen in chronic and acute renal failure are due to volume reduction during the diuretic phase.

5. _____ Acute renal failure normally progresses through three phases in the following order: oliguric, diuretic, and recovery phases.

6. _____ Oliguria refers to a urinary output of less than 400 mL/day, whereas anuria is a urinary output of less than 100 mL/day.

7. _____ Prerenal oliguria is a normal compensatory response of the kidney to reduced perfusion.

8. _____ Chronic kidney disease can be reversed, and total recovery of renal function is possible.

MULTIPLE CHOICE

Select the one best answer to each of the following questions.

9. Prerenal failure, regardless of the specific cause, has a single common etiologic factor, which is
   A. inactivation of the renal autoregulatory mechanisms.
   B. narrowing of afferent arterioles.
   C. a reduction in renal perfusion.
   D. a decreased effect of aldosterone and antidiuretic hormones.

10. All of the following could produce prerenal failure *except*
    A. myocardial infarction.
    B. pyelonephritis.
    C. septic shock.
    D. hemorrhage.

11. Damage to the kidney from nephrotoxic drugs
    A. is irreversible.
    B. impairs the epithelial cells of the renal tubules.
    C. impairs glomerular basement membrane permeability.
    D. commonly progresses to end-stage renal disease.

12. Back leakage of filtrate, an important aspect of the pathologic development of ATN,
    A. further reduces renal clearance of wastes.
    B. forces efferent and afferent arterioles to vasodilate.
    C. is due to dilation of renal tubules.
    D. increases platelet aggregation and the risk of thrombosis formation.

100

13. Acute renal failure produces all of the following characteristic alterations in laboratory values *except*
    A. elevated serum creatinine levels.
    B. azotemia.
    C. uremia.
    D. decreased serum potassium levels.

14. The clinical stage of chronic kidney disease known as "decreased renal reserve," or stage 1 to 2 disease,
    A. produces polyuria and nocturia.
    B. presents as mild azotemia.
    C. is asymptomatic.
    D. is characterized by elevated serum creatinine and BUN levels.

15. Findings associated with advanced chronic kidney disease but not likely to be found with acute renal failure include
    A. elevations in serum creatinine and BUN levels.
    B. fluid volume excess.
    C. hypocalcemia and anemia.
    D. metabolic acidosis.

16. The clinical stage of chronic kidney disease called "renal insufficiency," or stage 3 to 4 disease,
    A. may be controlled with dietary management.
    B. requires intervention with dialysis or renal transplantation.
    C. is associated with a nephron loss of about 50%.
    D. is successfully managed with diuretic therapy.

17. Which of the following patients is at highest risk for developing prerenal acute renal failure?
    A. An elderly patient with benign prostatic hyperplasia
    B. A young woman with acute pyelonephritis
    C. An elderly woman receiving nephrotoxic antibiotics
    D. A young man with significant postsurgical hemorrhage

18. Evidence-based interventions to slow the progression of chronic kidney disease include all of the following *except*
    A. blood glucose control for diabetic patients.
    B. blood pressure control.
    C. angiotensin-converting enzyme (ACE) inhibitors or angiotensin receptor blocker (ARB) drugs.
    D. a sodium-restricted diet.

19. Renal osteodystrophy develops as a complication of chronic kidney disease. The process is associated with
    A. hypercalcemia.
    B. hyperphosphatemia.
    C. hypoparathyroidism.
    D. hypokalemia.

20. The cause of death of most patients with chronic kidney disease is
    A. cardiovascular disease.
    B. kidney failure.
    C. malnutrition.
    D. volume overload.

Fill in the blanks with the appropriate word or words.

21. The primary risk factor for chronic kidney disease is _____ _____.

22. If prerenal renal failure is prolonged, it produces _____, which is one cause of acute tubular necrosis (ATN).

23. End-stage renal disease and uremia occur when more than _____% of nephrons are lost.

24. Patients with chronic kidney disease usually have a normocytic, normochromic anemia because of lack of _____.

25. Patients with chronic kidney disease who are being managed with diet may be asked to moderate their protein intake because protein is a source of _____ wastes and may worsen azotemia.

29 Disorders of the Lower Urinary Tract

TRUE/FALSE

Indicate whether the following statements are true (T) or false (F).

1. _____ Stress incontinence is due to inappropriate stimulation of the parasympathetic nervous system.

2. _____ Secretions from the prostate gland help to protect men from urinary tract infections.

3. _____ Stones forming in the urinary bladder are usually composed of calcium.

4. _____ Cystitis typically presents with dysuria, frequency, and urgency.

5. _____ Pregnant women with cystitis are carefully treated because of the increased risk of developing pyelonephritis.

6. _____ Spinal cord injury results in a loss of voluntary bladder control, called a neurogenic bladder.

7. _____ The normal residual urine volume in the adult bladder is up to 250 mL.

8. _____ Congenital anomalies of the lower urinary tract usually result in obstruction of urine flow.

9. _____ Primary cancers of the ureters or urethra are common.

10. _____ A common symptom of cystitis in children is bedwetting.

MULTIPLE CHOICE

Select the one best answer to each of the following questions.

11. Primary monosymptomatic nocturnal enuresis in children is
    A. always pathologic after the age of 5 years.
    B. nearly always managed with pharmacologic interventions.
    C. most commonly due to delayed maturation.
    D. frequently associated with daytime enuresis.

12. The most common cause of bladder calculi is
    A. urinary tract infection.
    B. urinary retention and stasis.
    C. increased dietary calcium intake.
    D. a reduced glomerular filtration rate (GFR).

13. Risk factors for the development of cystitis include all of the following *except*
    A. female gender.
    B. acidic urine.
    C. urinary stasis.
    D. diabetes mellitus.

14. Cystitis is
    A. an inflammation of the bladder lining.
    B. always associated with bacterial infection.
    C. a common cause of renal failure.
    D. always symptomatic.

103

15. Bladder tumors
   A. are most commonly formed in the musculature of the bladder wall.
   B. are always associated with exposure to carcinogens.
   C. are more common among African Americans.
   D. may present with occult or macroscopic hematuria.

16. Vesicoureteral reflux, a congenital malformation, is often diagnosed by
   A. a decreased frequency of voiding.
   B. an enlarged kidney found on an abdominal x-ray film.
   C. complaints of flank pain.
   D. an incidence of recurrent urinary tract infection.

17. The most common obstruction of the urinary tract found in children is ureteropelvic junction obstruction. This condition is
   A. more common in females.
   B. usually bilateral, affecting both ureters.
   C. usually diagnosed by ultrasound in utero.
   D. likely to require surgical intervention.

18. Congenital malformations of the ureters primarily produce signs and symptoms related to
   A. abnormal bladder distention.
   B. elevations in blood urea nitrogen (BUN) and serum creatinine levels.
   C. urinary stasis.
   D. renal atrophy.

19. The most common manifestation of bladder cancer is
   A. urgency.
   B. hematuria.
   C. frequency.
   D. dysuria.

20. The most common cause of cystitis is
   A. *Escherichia coli.*
   B. organisms associated with sexually transmitted infections.
   C. fungal organisms.
   D. viral organisms.

21. The primary risk factor for bladder cancer is
   A. smoking.
   B. air pollution.
   C. family history.
   D. infection.

FILL IN THE BLANKS

Fill in the blanks with the appropriate word or words.

22. Bladder contraction is controlled by the _____ _____ _____.

23. A dilation of the distal ureters is called a _____.

24. A chronic illness with no known cause that causes bladder pain, and often urgency, frequency, and nocturia, is called

   _____ _____.

25. An overactive detrusor muscle is the cause of _____ incontinence.

26. Ureteral irritation by urolithiasis usually results in the clinical signs of pain and _____.

27. The external sphincter of the bladder is controlled by the _____ _____ _____.

28. Bedridden or confused elderly patients may experience _____ incontinence.

29. If urine culture is done, then antibiotic therapy is guided by the results of _____ testing.

30. Children who have recurring urinary tract infections or pyelonephritis should be evaluated for _____ defects of the urinary tract.

UNIT VIII: Case Studies

T.G. arrives at the nurse practitioner clinic complaining of a burning sensation during urination, as well as a feeling of needing to urinate more often than usual. She is a 25-year-old graduate student and has recently returned from her honeymoon.

1. The symptoms T.G. reports are characteristic of
   A. a bladder tumor.
   B. pyelonephritis.
   C. bladder calculi.
   D. cystitis.

2. In order to confirm the diagnosis, the nurse practitioner orders
   A. a urinalysis.
   B. an intravenous pyelogram.
   C. an abdominal x-ray.
   D. an abdominal ultrasound.

3. Results of this diagnostic test that support the preliminary diagnosis would be
   A. radiopaque stones visible in the bladder.
   B. obstructed renal perfusion.
   C. bacteria in the urine.
   D. an abdominal mass.

4. The appropriate intervention for the nurse practitioner to initiate would be
   A. a standard course of antibiotic therapy.
   B. renal ultrasound to evaluate for pyelonephritis.
   C. referral to a surgeon.
   D. referral to a nephrologist.

5. Counseling that the nurse practitioner would provide for T.G. would also likely include all of the following *except*
   A. increased fluid intake.
   B. abstinence from sexual intercourse.
   C. urination following sexual intercourse.
   D. correct cleansing technique following bowel movements.

Sixty-five-year-old C.V. was admitted to the hospital for management of dehydration associated with a severe gastrointestinal flu.

6. For which type of acute renal failure is C.V. at risk?
   A. Prerenal renal failure
   B. Postrenal renal failure
   C. Pyelonephritis
   D. Glomerulonephritis

7. C.V. develops prerenal oliguria. Which of the following would *not* be found among her laboratory results?
    A. Low urinary sodium levels
    B. A BUN to creatinine ratio greater than 20:1
    C. A low urine specific gravity
    D. A high urine osmolality

8. The appropriate intervention for the prerenal oliguria phase of C.V.'s disorder would be
    A. dialysis.
    B. extracellular volume expansion.
    C. monitoring the serum BUN level and limiting protein intake.
    D. aggressive diuretic therapy.

9. C.V. responds poorly to therapy and enters the oliguric phase of acute renal failure. When this occurs,
    A. tubular casts may be found in the urine.
    B. hematuria may ensue.
    C. an increase in urinary output is expected.
    D. the concentration of sodium in the urine declines.

10. Improvement in C.V.'s GFR correlates most closely with
    A. normalizing of serum creatinine levels.
    B. normalizing of BUN levels.
    C. normalizing of the urine specific gravity.
    D. normalizing of albumin levels.

A.P. is a 56-year-old man being treated for chronic pyelonephritis. He is currently living in a homeless shelter, but when the weather warms in the spring, he typically "moves outside somewhere."

11. The cause of chronic pyelonephritis is
    A. prostatic hypertrophy.
    B. glomerulonephritis.
    C. recurrent urinary infections.
    D. failure to respond to the urge to void.

12. The health care workers are concerned about A.P. because chronic pyelonephritis is
    A. a premalignant condition.
    B. a common cause of cystitis.
    C. a cause of significant fluid and electrolyte abnormalities.
    D. a leading cause of renal failure.

13. Careful, thorough teaching will be necessary because
    A. A.P. is not likely to have access to hygienic bathroom facilities.
    B. a balanced diet and increased protein intake are essential.
    C. A.P. is not likely to void on a regular basis.
    D. antibiotic therapy must be continued for a prolonged course.

14. Compare and contrast cystitis and pyelonephritis by filling in the following table. Write "yes" or "no" in the appropriate columns.

Characteristic	Cystitis	Pyelonephritis
Frequency, urgency, and dysuria		
Increased serum white blood cells		
Flank pain		
Fever		
Costovertebral angle tenderness		
Urinary casts		

Arriving at the emergency department in acute pain, 20-year-old M.N. is close to tears. He says the pain began when he was sitting in his college class, nearly causing him to double over. He tells the triage nurse that it "just came on—bang, and it just gets worse." He rates his pain as 10 out of 10, stating that it is located low and to the left of his spine. It seems to "come in waves."

15. M.N.'s description is classic for renal colic associated with calculi. Other associated signs or symptoms of calculi typically include
    A. nausea and vomiting.
    B. decreased urinary output.
    C. enuresis.
    D. diarrhea.

16. Most renal calculi are initially evaluated with which of the following diagnostic tests?
    A. Urine culture
    B. X-ray film of the kidneys, ureters, and bladder
    C. Serum creatinine and BUN levels
    D. Computed tomography (CT) scan

17. It is determined that M.N.'s calculi are small (<5 mm) and so should pass in his urine. Treatment at this time will include
    A. bed rest.
    B. hospitalization and intravenous fluids.
    C. nothing by mouth (NPO) and giving antiemetics.
    D. pain medication and increased fluids.

Seven-year-old L.E. has developed acute glomerulonephritis following a severe throat infection. Fortunately, he was a healthy boy before this, so his physician and family are optimistic that he will make a full recovery.

18. If acute glomerulonephritis progresses to acute renal failure, which type will it cause?
    A. Prerenal renal failure
    B. Intrarenal renal failure
    C. Acute tubular necrosis (ATN)
    D. Postrenal renal failure

19. L.E. begins to have significant proteinuria, and a 24-hour urine collection contains 4 g of protein. L.E. has progressed to
    A. renal failure.
    B. ATN.
    C. needing dialysis.
    D. nephrotic syndrome.

20. The loss of significant protein in the urine contributes to all of the following manifestations *except*
    A. edema.
    B. ascites.
    C. hematuria.
    D. effusions in the pleural space.

21. All forms of acute glomerulonephritis share the same basic pathophysiology, which is
    A. damage to efferent arterioles.
    B. tubular epithelial sloughing.
    C. glomerular inflammation.
    D. glomerular epithelial cell apoptosis.

The nurses working in the outpatient hemodialysis unit are very familiar with B.J. He has been receiving dialysis treatments for end-stage kidney disease three times per week for 4 years. He is 44 years old and works as an accountant. The cause of his chronic kidney disease is diabetes, which he has had since he was 11 years old.

22. When B.J. comes in for treatment, he usually has some of the signs and symptoms of fluid volume overload (especially if he ate potato chips the night before!). All of the following would be seen *except*
    A. crackles in the bases of the lungs.
    B. 2+ edema of the ankles.
    C. jugular venous distention.
    D. weak peripheral pulses.

23. Patients with chronic renal failure usually exhibit
    A. bradycardia.
    B. hypokalemia.
    C. hypocalcemia.
    D. hematomas.

24. B.J. is at risk for some problems because of his chronic kidney disease that are not found with acute renal failure. These include
    A. osteodystrophy.
    B. metabolic acidosis.
    C. elevated serum potassium.
    D. azotemia.

25. Chronic kidney disease is
    A. a reversible disorder.
    B. a progressive disorder.
    C. a disorder with an unpredictable course.
    D. a disorder that spontaneously improves with time.

26. The diet of a patient in end-stage kidney disease usually is restricted in all of the following *except*
    A. fluid.
    B. potassium.
    C. phosphate.
    D. calories.

30 Male Genital and Reproductive Function

MATCHING

1. Match each of the following anatomic terms with the appropriate letter in the figure.

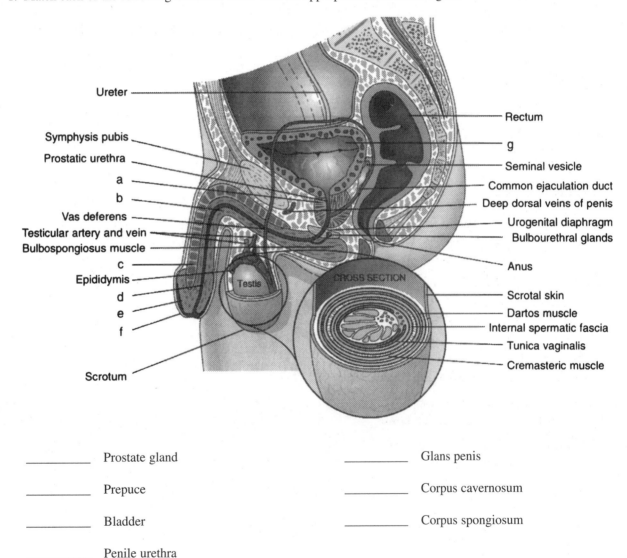

_____ Prostate gland

_____ Prepuce

_____ Bladder

_____ Penile urethra

_____ Glans penis

_____ Corpus cavernosum

_____ Corpus spongiosum

TRUE/FALSE

Indicate whether the following statements are true (T) or false (F).

2. _____ Movement of urine through the ureters is facilitated by smooth muscle contractions.

3. _____ The epididymis is the area of the testes where sperm are produced.

4. _____ Penile erection is mediated primarily by the sympathetic nervous system.

5. _____ External genitalia development, differentiating male from female, begins at the sixth week of fetal life.

6. _____ The normal adult male bladder capacity is 450 to 500 mL.

7. _____ Sertoli cells in the testes produce testosterone.

8. _____ The epididymis originates in the testes and terminates in the seminal vesicles.

9. _____ Gonadotropin-releasing hormone is released from the hypothalamus.

10. _____ Both males and females synthesize and release luteinizing hormone (LH) and follicle-stimulating hormone (FSH) from the anterior pituitary.

MULTIPLE CHOICE

Select the one best answer to each of the following questions.

11. All of the following are involved in providing components for the seminal fluid *except*
    A. the prostate gland.
    B. the bladder.
    C. the seminal vesicles.
    D. the bulbourethral glands.

12. The Leydig cells of the testes
    A. maintain testicular temperature.
    B. produce sperm.
    C. secrete testosterone.
    D. are part of the immune system.

13. Which of the following is a characteristic of spermatozoa?
    A. They contain 23 chromosomes.
    B. Their development is solely through mitotic reproduction.
    C. They are fully mature in a few hours.
    D. They produce energy through aerobic metabolism.

14. All of the following changes occur in male reproduction with aging *except*
    A. the number of sperm produced decreases.
    B. the penis becomes smaller.
    C. the testes hypertrophy.
    D. testosterone production declines.

15. Only 10% of the total ejaculate volume is composed of sperm, but men must have a high sperm count for fertilization because
    A. multiple sperm must simultaneously enter the egg.
    B. most sperm are unable to survive following ejaculation.
    C. immature sperm make up most of the ejaculate.
    D. multiple cellular layers of the egg must be penetrated.

16. Negative feedback from the testes to the hypothalamus to regulate gonadotropin-releasing hormone is provided by
    A. testosterone.
    B. cortisol.
    C. growth hormone.
    D. Sertoli factor.

17. Inhibin is a hormone that
    A. is produced by Leydig cells in the testes.
    B. inhibits pituitary release of gonadotropins.
    C. stimulates growth of secondary sex characteristics.
    D. stimulates sperm production.

18. Sperm become activated after being exposed to vaginal fluids. This activation process is called
    A. fertilization.
    B. acrosome excitation.
    C. capacitation.
    D. spermaticalization.

31 Alterations in Male Genital and Reproductive Function

Select the one best answer to each of the following questions.

1. The most common site of urinary obstruction in male newborns and infants is
   A. where the ureters enter the bladder wall.
   B. at the urethral valves in the distal prostatic urethra.
   C. at the urethral meatus.
   D. where the renal pelvis empties into the ureter.

2. In hypospadias, the urethral meatus is located
   A. on the ventral surface of the penis or on the perineum.
   B. on the dorsal surface of the penis near the glans.
   C. immediately anterior to the anus.
   D. midway on the shaft of the penis.

3. A persistent, painful erection is called
   A. epispadias.
   B. paraphimosis.
   C. resistant.
   D. priapism.

4. Secondary erectile dysfunction may be caused by
   A. psychiatric problems.
   B. diabetes mellitus.
   C. vascular trauma to the penis in childhood.
   D. excessive sympathetic innervation.

5. A diagnosis of cryptorchidism increases the risk for developing
   A. penile cancer.
   B. prostatitis.
   C. testicular cancer.
   D. erectile dysfunction.

6. Testicular torsion can result in
   A. hydrocele.
   B. testicular cancer.
   C. spermatocele.
   D. testicular death.

7. A patient presenting with a bladder infection and a swollen, red, and tender scrotum would probably be diagnosed as having
   A. syphilis.
   B. genital herpes.
   C. epididymitis.
   D. cystocele.

8. A decrease in the diameter and force of the urinary stream plus difficulty in initiating urination with dribbling at the conclusion of the void are common presenting signs and symptoms of
   A. benign prostatic hyperplasia (BPH).
   B. prostatitis.
   C. hydrocele.
   D. urinary tract infection.

9. All of the following statements regarding prostate cancer are true *except*
   A. an elevated serum prostate-specific antigen (PSA) level may be indicative.
   B. therapy always includes surgical intervention.
   C. bone and lungs are typical sites of metastasis.
   D. the risk of development increases with age.

10. Micropenis is
    A. not diagnosed until a boy has entered puberty.
    B. always associated with multiple other anomalies of the genitourinary system.
    C. not amenable to treatment interventions.
    D. usually due to a testosterone production abnormality.

TRUE/FALSE

Indicate whether the following statements are true (T) or false (F).

11. _____ Penile cancer is rare.

12. _____ Most cases of erectile dysfunction have a secondary cause.

13. _____ BPH is a risk factor for prostate cancer.

14. _____ In paraphimosis, the foreskin cannot be retracted from the glans, whereas with phimosis, the foreskin that has been retracted cannot be repositioned over the glans.

15. _____ The cause of hypospadias is an error in the fetal development of the male external genitalia.

FILL IN THE BLANKS

Fill in the blanks with the appropriate word or words.

16. Differentiation of primitive gonadal tissues into ovaries and testes begins during the _____ week of gestation.

17. Epididymitis is most frequently caused by _____.

18. The organism most commonly responsible for prostatitis is _____ _____.

19. Erectile dysfunction is often attributed to drugs that interfere with autonomic function, such as _____.

20. A low male libido is associated with _____ deficiency.

21. An elderly male with _____ _____ has a curvature of the penis caused by plaque formation on the corpora cavernosa.

22. Erectile dysfunction is a common disorder in aging men and also those taking certain medications and those with

    _____.

23. Many patients with erectile dysfunction are helped by medications that temporarily increase blood flow to the penis because they inhibit _____ resulting in an increase of cyclic guanosine monophosphate (cGMP).

24. Men with low sperm count are likely to have _____.

25. Approximately _____ percent of men over 60 years of age have benign prostatic hyperplasia and an enlarged prostate.

32 Female Genital and Reproductive Function

MATCHING

1. Match each of the following anatomic terms with the appropriate letter in the figure:

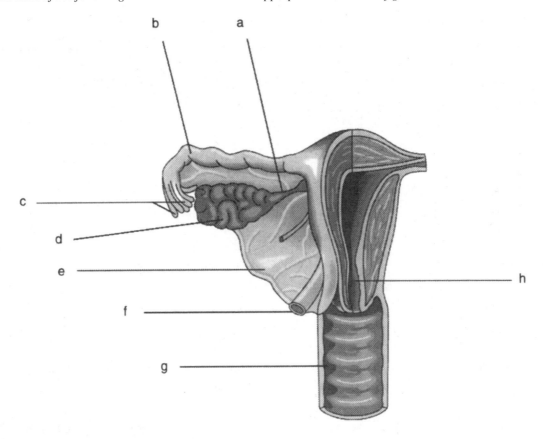

_____ Fallopian tube   _____ Fimbria

_____ Broad ligament   _____ Ovarian ligament

_____ Uterus   _____ Vagina

_____ Ovary   _____ Uterosacral ligament

Match each definition on the left with its term on the right. Not all terms are defined.

2. _____ Muscular area where the ureters enter the bladder

3. _____ Stimulates testosterone synthesis

4. _____ Responsible for stimulating ovulation

5. _____ Secreted by the corpus luteum

6. _____ In addition to estrogen and progesterone, these stimulate breast development at puberty

7. _____ Site of fertilization of the ovum by sperm

8. _____ Hormone responsible for stimulating uterine contractions of labor

9. _____ Secreted by the placenta to assist in maintaining pregnancy

10. _____ The time in pregnancy when fetal movement can be felt

A. Detrusor
B. First trimester
C. Trigone
D. Uterus
E. Follicle-stimulating hormone (FSH) and luteinizing hormone (LH)
F. Fallopian tube
G. Human chorionic gonadotropin
H. Second trimester
I. Testosterone
J. LH
K. Growth hormone and prolactin
L. Oxytocin
M. Estrogen and progesterone

TRUE/FALSE

Indicate whether the following statements are true (T) or false (F).

11. _____ Endometrial proliferation is enhanced by the hormone progesterone.

12. _____ Release of milk from the breast tissue ducts is mediated by oxytocin from the posterior pituitary gland.

13. _____ One maternal change that occurs during pregnancy is an increase in blood volume of 1 to 2 L.

14. _____ Menopause occurs because of a decrease in the number of ovarian follicles.

15. _____ The greatest fetal growth occurs during the first trimester.

16. _____ All ovarian eggs (oogonia) are present at birth; no more are developed following birth.

17. _____ Lymphatic drainage of the breast tissue is predominantly into nodes located near the diaphragm.

FILL IN THE BLANKS

Fill in the blanks with the appropriate word or words.

18. The _____ is the inner layer of uterine tissue that proliferates and is then sloughed during menstruation.

19. The decline in estrogen associated with menopause may contribute to _____, which increases a woman's risk for fractures.

20. Transient nausea is most common in the _____ trimester of pregnancy.

33 Alterations in Female Genital and Reproductive Function

MATCHING

Match each definition on the left with its term on the right.

1. _____ the presence of endometrial tissue outside of the uterine lining.

2. _____ widespread infection affecting multiple pelvic organs.

3. _____ benign fibroid growths in the uterine muscle.

4. _____ protrusion of the rectal wall into posterior wall of the vagina

5. _____ abnormally painful menstruation.

A. Leiomyoma
B. Endometriosis
C. Pelvic inflammatory disease
D. Dysmenorrhea
E. Rectocele

MULTIPLE CHOICE

Select the one best answer to each of the following questions.

6. Amenorrhea is primarily associated with alterations in the quantity or action of
   A. progesterone.
   B. estrogen.
   C. luteinizing hormone (LH).
   D. follicle-stimulating hormone (FSH).

7. The presence of endometrial polyps or endometrial hyperplasia is a common cause of
   A. metrorrhagia.
   B. menorrhagia.
   C. hypomenorrhea.
   D. polymenorrhea.

8. The symptoms of dysmenorrhea
   A. are a reflection of a neurosis.
   B. are associated with an abnormal amount of menstrual bleeding.
   C. typically increase with age.
   D. can be reduced with drugs that inhibit prostaglandin formation.

9. Uterine prolapse, cystocele, and rectocele may all be the result of
   A. repeated infections.
   B. chronic constipation.
   C. hormonal abnormalities.
   D. pregnancy and childbirth.

10. Pelvic inflammatory disease is managed aggressively because long-term effects can include
    A. preterm labor.
    B. renal failure.
    C. infertility.
    D. transmission to the fetus.

11. Uterine leiomyomas (fibroids) tend to decrease after menopause because their growth appears to be dependent on
    A. estrogen.
    B. progesterone.
    C. prolactin.
    D. testosterone.

12. Endometriosis is associated with
    A. frequent episodes of pelvic inflammatory disease.
    B. minimal discomfort.
    C. reduced fertility rates.
    D. fluid-filled sacs attached to the endometrial wall.

13. Early-stage cervical cancer may be detected by
    A. thick gray discharge into the vagina.
    B. abnormal Papanicolaou (Pap) test results.
    C. development of abnormal uterine bleeding.
    D. symptoms of urinary tract infection.

14. Fibrocystic breast disease is characterized by
    A. an increased risk of breast cancer.
    B. benign neoplastic growths in breast tissue.
    C. a decreased ability to breast feed offspring.
    D. breast masses that present on a cyclic basis and are tender to palpation.

15. The primary risk factor for breast cancer is
    A. decreased estrogen.
    B. increasing age.
    C. multiparity.
    D. dietary patterns.

FILL IN THE BLANKS

Fill in the blanks with the appropriate word or words.

16. Protrusion of the bladder wall into the vagina is called a _____ and is most often due to _____.

17. Pregnancy-induced hypertension can be screened for by monitoring blood pressure and testing the urine for

    _____.

18. Although how it is done remains controversial, _____ intervention is the primary approach to breast cancer.

19. Cervical cancer in its earliest, in situ, stage is diagnosed by the _____ test.

20. Most breast cancers occur in the _____ _____ quadrant of the breast.

34 Sexually Transmitted Infections

Select the one best answer to each of the following questions.

1. Many sexually transmitted infections can also be contracted by
   A. a vaginally delivered newborn of an infected mother.
   B. ingestion of contaminated food.
   C. handling of infected material.
   D. inhalation of airborne spores.

2. A patient suspected of having a sexually transmitted infection who presents with inflammation of the urethra or uterine cervix and/or signs and symptoms of pelvic inflammatory disease most likely is infected with
   A. *Neisseria gonorrhoeae.*
   B. *Treponema pallidum.*
   C. herpesvirus.
   D. *Haemophilus ducreyi.*

3. The sexually transmitted infection that presents with formation of a painless ulcer (called a chancre) and later progresses to a systemic form is
   A. herpes.
   B. chlamydial infection.
   C. syphilis.
   D. hepatitis B.

4. Herpesvirus type 2 may remain in the body in a latent form. Exacerbations of the infection are commonly triggered by
   A. reinfection.
   B. sexual intercourse.
   C. temperature extremes.
   D. emotional stress.

5. Which of the following statements about genital warts (*Condylomata acuminata*) is *false*?
   A. They are highly contagious.
   B. They are rarely visible because the growths develop deep in tissues.
   C. They are due to infection with a type of human papillomavirus.
   D. They have an incubation period averaging 4 months.

6. In women, gonorrhea is usually
   A. less common than among men.
   B. associated with a rash on the torso.
   C. slower to incubate.
   D. asymptomatic.

7. Late, tertiary syphilis can result in all of the following changes in the central nervous system *except*
   A. blindness.
   B. motor weakness.
   C. hearing loss.
   D. decreased mental functioning.

8. If untreated, lymphogranuloma venereum abscesses due to chlamydial infection
   A. are walled into granulomas.
   B. may form fistulas.
   C. are absorbed deeper into the body.
   D. may become gangrenous.

FILL IN THE BLANKS

Fill in the blanks with the appropriate word or words.

9. Transmission of *Chlamydia* during childbirth can result in an infection of the _____ of the newborn.

10. Inflammation of the fallopian tubes is called _____.

11. The type of herpesvirus responsible for infections in the genital, anal, and perianal region is herpes simplex virus (HSV) type _____.

12. Primary syphilis lesions left untreated will spontaneously resolve in _____ to _____ _____.

13. The vaccine developed to prevent cervical cancer associated with the human papillomavirus (HPV) also reduces the risk of developing _____ _____.

14. The majority of sexually transmitted infections are due to the _____ family of organisms.

15. Herpetic infections are especially serious for those who are _____.

UNIT IX: Case Studies

I.L. is a healthy 28-year-old woman who is pregnant with her first child. A nursing student is visiting her and her husband. The student's primary responsibility is to identify learning needs and design teaching plans to address those needs. I.L. and her husband are fascinated with the changes in her body and learning about the development of the fetus.

1. "I understand that the placenta is responsible for bringing oxygen and nutrients to the fetus, but does it serve any other function?" asks I.L. The student would be correct in responding
   A. "Yes, it also secretes hormones that increase the size of the uterus and make structures more elastic for delivery."
   B. "No, that is the only function that the placenta performs."
   C. "Yes, it stabilizes the embryo when it is very small so that it cannot leave the uterus."
   D. "Yes, it secretes hormones that maintain the mother's health during pregnancy."

2. In response to I.L.'s question about weight gain during pregnancy, the student would be correct in basing a reply on the fact that
   A. most of the weight gain occurs in the second and third trimesters.
   B. the average weight gain in pregnancy is 35 pounds.
   C. the weight of the fetus constitutes most of the total weight gain.
   D. most of the weight gained, beyond the weight of the fetus, is attributable to edema fluid.

3. The student tells I.L. that all of the following changes in her body would be normal *except*
   A. breasts doubling in size.
   B. an increase in the respiratory rate.
   C. a slight elevation in temperature.
   D. swelling of the face, especially around the eyes.

120

Chapter **34** Sexually Transmitted Infections

Copyright © 2019, Elsevier Inc. All rights reserved.

4. The primary vitamin or mineral a pregnant woman needs, because stored levels are not sufficient to meet the maternal and fetal needs, is
   A. calcium.
   B. vitamin C.
   C. iron.
   D. magnesium.

F.R. is 47 years old and has come to see her physician for her annual physical. During their conversation, F.R. describes a menstrual pattern that has been irregular over the past few months. She wonders if she might be experiencing menopause.

5. Additional signs or symptoms of menopause may include
   A. increased frequency of urination.
   B. sudden sensations of warmth of the neck and face.
   C. a clear, thick discharge from the vagina.
   D. muscle aches.

6. The underlying cause of menopause is
   A. sealing of the cervix.
   B. structural changes in the uterus.
   C. estrogen deficiency.
   D. progesterone excess.

7. The changes associated with perimenopause and menopause increase the risk for
   A. lung diseases such as asthma.
   B. osteoporosis.
   C. autoimmune diseases.
   D. type 2 diabetes.

A 19-year-old female student comes to the Student Health Center complaining of painful urination and suspects a urinary tract infection. A laboratory analysis report indicates a gonococcal infection.

8. In women, gonorrhea
   A. is uncommon.
   B. has no effect on later reproduction.
   C. usually has no symptoms.
   D. always coexists with *Chlamydia trachomatis* infection.

9. In men, gonorrhea
   A. usually has no symptoms.
   B. frequently causes urinary tract infection.
   C. may cause inflammation of the Bartholin glands.
   D. may result in epididymitis.

10. In patients with symptomatic gonorrhea, the infection may cause inflammation of the
    A. pharynx.
    B. retina.
    C. joints.
    D. heart valves.

B.H. is a 53-year-old woman who discovered a lump in her breast while performing breast self-examination. Upon seeing her physician and having a mammogram and biopsy, she is convinced that she has a carcinoma of the breast.

11. A major difference found on breast self-examination between malignant and benign growths in the breast is that malignant growths are
    A. smaller.
    B. nontender.
    C. somewhat movable.
    D. softer to the touch.

12. A review of B.H.'s history reveals which of the following as a significant risk factor for breast cancer?
    A. Onset of menses at age 13 years and menopause at age 50 years
    B. A mother with breast cancer
    C. A history of fibrocystic breast disease
    D. A diet averaging 20% fat

13. The most common location for malignant tumors of the breast is the
    A. nipple area.
    B. inner aspect, near the sternum.
    C. lower surface.
    D. upper, outer quadrant.

14. The prognosis for breast cancer is most contingent on
    A. the size of the tumor.
    B. the location of the tumor in the breast.
    C. the age of the woman.
    D. the degree of lymph node involvement.

Sixty-five-year-old D.E. comes to see his physician with complaints of difficulty initiating his urinary stream and dribbling after voiding. He has postponed this physician's appointment out of fear that he might have prostate cancer. Recently, however, he began to have frequency, urgency, and some dysuria, so he followed through with the appointment; he is still very worried. His physician performs a rectal examination to evaluate the prostate.

15. The prostate examination reveals an enlargement. A prostate-specific antigen (PSA) test is ordered and shows that the PSA level is normal. These findings are indicative of
    A. prostate cancer.
    B. benign prostatic hyperplasia (BPH).
    C. prostatic obstruction.
    D. the absence of any pathologic process.

16. The symptoms of urinary tract infection in the presence of an enlarged, painless prostate gland are most characteristic of
    A. Peyronie disease.
    B. prostatitis.
    C. BPH.
    D. any condition affecting the prostate gland.

17. The primary etiologic factor associated with the development of BPH appears to be
    A. recurrent infection.
    B. a viral infection elsewhere in the body.
    C. increasing age of the male genitourinary system.
    D. urinary retention.

35 Gastrointestinal Function

MATCHING

1. *Match each of the following anatomic terms with its appropriate letter in the figure.*

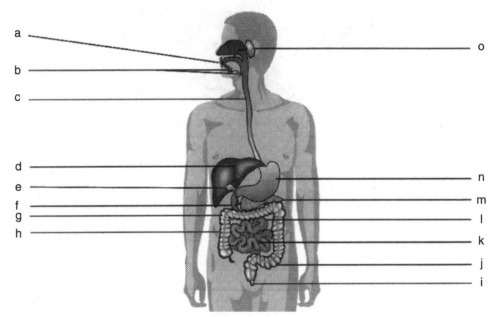

_____ Anus		_____ Descending colon	
_____ Liver		_____ Parotid glands	
_____ Ascending colon		_____ Duodenum	
_____ Mouth		_____ Pancreas	
_____ Esophagus		_____ Ileum	
_____ Salivary glands		_____ Transverse colon	
_____ Gallbladder		_____ Jejunum	
_____ Stomach			

2. *Match each of the following anatomic terms with its appropriate letter in the figure.*

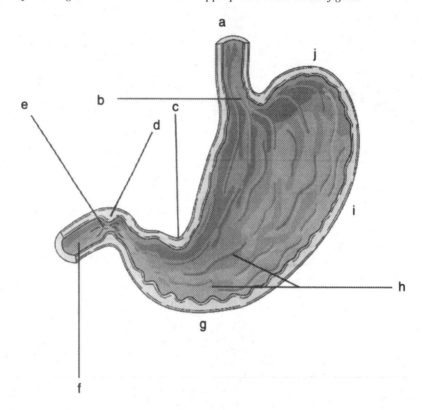

_____	Angular notch	_____	Pyloric sphincter
_____	Esophagus	_____	Cardia
_____	Antrum	_____	Pylorus
_____	Fundus	_____	Duodenum
_____	Body	_____	Rugae

Match the enzyme on the left with the type of nutrient it cleaves on the right. Answers may be used more than once.

3. _____ Chymotrypsin

4. _____ Trypsin

5. _____ Lipase

6. _____ α-Amylase

7. _____ Pepsin

8. _____ Sucrase

9. _____ Lactase

10. _____ Maltase

11. _____ Aminopeptidase

12. _____ Carboxypeptidase

A. Fats
B. Proteins
C. Carbohydrates

124

TRUE/FALSE

Indicate whether the following statements are true (T) or false (F).

13. _____ The intrinsic nervous system of the gastrointestinal tract has a more direct role in the control of GI functions than does the autonomic nervous system.

14. _____ Secretion of bile from the gallbladder is stimulated by gastrin release into the stomach.

15. _____ If the contents of the duodenum are acidic or hypertonic, gastric emptying may be slowed.

16. _____ Parasympathetic stimulation of the large bowel produces increased motility.

17. _____ Propulsion of gastrointestinal contents is primarily regulated by the autonomic nervous system.

18. _____ The vomiting center is located in the central nervous system.

19. _____ Parietal cells of the stomach secrete pepsinogen, which is activated to pepsin in the presence of intrinsic factor.

20. _____ Digestion of protein is initiated by the release of amylase into the duodenum by the pancreas.

21. _____ No digestion of dietary fats occurs until the fats reach the small intestine.

22. _____ The primary site of nutrient and water absorption is the small intestine.

23. _____ Unlike fat or carbohydrate digestion, protein digestion begins in the stomach.

24. _____ Fat emulsification involves the enzymatic breakdown of large lipid molecules by bile.

25. _____ Water absorption from the gastrointestinal tract occurs via active transport systems.

26. _____ The lower esophageal sphincter (LES) will not release food into the stomach until the food has been fully processed by salivary digestive enzymes.

27. _____ Babies younger than 3 to 4 months are usually fed only liquids because their enzyme systems are too immature to break down solid foods.

28. _____ The secretory and absorptive functions of the intestine are not fully mature for the first 2 years of life.

29. _____ Decreased intake in the elderly is most commonly a result of a reduced basal metabolic rate.

30. _____ Intestinal transit time increases with age, increasing the risk for constipation in the elderly.

36 Gastrointestinal Disorders

COMPARE/CONTRAST

1. *Compare and contrast the inflammatory bowel diseases ulcerative colitis and Crohn disease by filling in "yes" or "no" in the appropriate column.*

Characteristic	Ulcerative Colitis	Crohn Disease
Abscess formation		
Bloody diarrhea		
Fistula formation		
Rectal bleeding		
Mucosal layer involvement		
Transmural involvement		

FILL IN THE BLANKS

Fill in the blanks with the appropriate word or words.

2. A common cause of constipation is a _____ _____ diet.

3. In Western countries, acute gastritis is most commonly associated with the overuse of _____, _____,

   and _____.

4. _____ ulcers usually cause pain when the stomach is empty or shortly after eating, whereas _____
   ulcers cause pain 2 to 3 hours after eating.

5. Conditions that may result in mechanical bowel obstruction include _____, which is a twisted bowel, and

   _____, in which the bowel telescopes upon itself.

6. An acquired bowel disease that may develop at any age, _____ is most often caused by prolonged constipation.

MULTIPLE CHOICE

Select the one best answer to each of the following questions.

7. All of the following may result in dysphagia *except*
   A. altered neuromuscular ability to coordinate movement of material to the esophagus.
   B. impaired relaxation of the lower esophageal sphincter (LES).
   C. decreased peristalsis of the distal portion of the esophagus.
   D. excessive production of stomach acid.

8. Abdominal pain that manifests as visceral pain is characterized by
   A. pain at the umbilicus.
   B. being extremely sharp and well localized.
   C. diaphragmatic or peritoneal involvement.
   D. being diffuse and poorly localized, with a cramping or burning sensation.

126

9. The diarrhea seen with inflammatory bowel disease is primarily an example of
    A. osmotic diarrhea.
    B. secretory diarrhea.
    C. exudative diarrhea.
    D. diarrhea due to increased motility.

10. A common cause of stomatitis seen in immunosuppressed patients is
    A. *Candida albicans* infection.
    B. vitamin deficiency.
    C. exposure to chemical irritants.
    D. gastroesophageal reflux.

11. Mallory-Weiss syndrome usually is caused by
    A. a hiatal hernia.
    B. overdosage with acetaminophen.
    C. cirrhosis.
    D. a severe vomiting episode.

12. Risk factors for gastroesophageal reflux include
    A. a hiatal hernia.
    B. constipation.
    C. esophagitis.
    D. decreased gastric acidity.

13. *Helicobacter pylori* infection has been implicated in all of the following *except*
    A. chronic gastritis.
    B. gastric cancer.
    C. peptic ulcer disease (PUD).
    D. acute gastritis.

14. Common manifestations of PUD include
    A. diarrhea.
    B. burning epigastric pain.
    C. vomiting.
    D. bright red blood in the stool.

15. A patient with PUD should be encouraged to avoid
    A. high-fiber foods.
    B. aspirin and nonsteroidal antiinflammatory drugs (NSAIDs).
    C. excessive intake of liquids.
    D. lying down immediately after eating.

16. A major predisposing factor to the development of pseudomembranous enterocolitis is
    A. a history of inflammatory bowel disease.
    B. intestinal hypoxia.
    C. antibiotic therapy.
    D. contaminated foods.

17. The primary life-threatening complication of appendicitis is
    A. peritonitis.
    B. dehydration.
    C. cardiac arrest.
    D. abscess formation.

18. Which of the following is a *true* statement regarding diverticular disease?
    A. It can occur anywhere in the gastrointestinal tract.
    B. It most frequently affects young adults.
    C. If diverticuli become inflamed, intestinal obstruction may result.
    D. The condition is most common among societies where the diet is high in cellulose.

19. All of the following could result in a *mechanical* bowel obstruction *except*
    A. volvulus.
    B. intussusception.
    C. adhesions.
    D. narcotic analgesic administration.

20. The manifestations of bowel obstruction are related to
    A. decreased absorption of nutrients.
    B. accumulation of fluid and gas proximal to the obstruction.
    C. edema impairing biliary secretion.
    D. the death of intestinal bacteria.

21. A congenital condition of the colon in which there are insufficient autonomic ganglia in the bowel resulting in contraction but inadequate relaxation to move the fecal mass forward efficiently is called
    A. short-bowel syndrome.
    B. celiac disease.
    C. irritable bowel syndrome.
    D. Hirschsprung disease.

22. Malabsorption of nutrients is secondary to
    A. inadequate nutrient intake.
    B. peristaltic dysfunction.
    C. conditions that affect the colon.
    D. conditions that affect the small intestine.

23. Carcinoma of the stomach is
    A. slow growing and therefore highly curable with early diagnosis.
    B. associated with precancerous polyps.
    C. correlated with *H. pylori* infection.
    D. primarily managed with chemotherapy.

24. Warning signs for colon cancer include
    A. blood in the stool.
    B. epigastric pain.
    C. nausea or vomiting after meals.
    D. loss of appetite.

25. Constipation is defined as fewer than _____ stools per week.
    A. one
    B. two
    C. three
    D. four

26. Acute gastroenteritis usually is caused by
    A. stress.
    B. spicy foods.
    C. overeating.
    D. infectious agents.

37 Alterations in Function of the Gallbladder and Exocrine Pancreas

Select the one best answer to each of the following questions.

1. Risk factors for gallstone formation include all of the following *except*
   A. female gender.
   B. cystic fibrosis.
   C. gastritis.
   D. obesity.

2. Patients with acute pancreatitis are closely monitored for the development of the potentially lethal complication of
   A. pancreatic rupture.
   B. circulatory shock.
   C. cardiac dysrhythmias.
   D. stroke.

3. Like acute pancreatitis, the development of chronic pancreatitis is most frequently associated with
   A. biliary disease.
   B. diabetes.
   C. alcohol abuse.
   D. malnutrition.

4. A gallbladder attack is most often characterized by
   A. left upper quadrant pain.
   B. pain recurring in 5- to 10-minute cycles.
   C. pain with nausea and bloating.
   D. steatorrhea.

5. Chronic pancreatitis can result in all of the following *except*
   A. malabsorption.
   B. diabetes mellitus.
   C. inflammatory bowel disease.
   D. pseudocyst formation.

6. Chronic pancreatitis disrupts the organ's exocrine functions. Therapy for this condition involves digestive enzyme supplementation and
   A. a low-fat diet.
   B. insulin replacement.
   C. glucagon supplementation.
   D. fat-soluble vitamins.

7. The pancreas has both endocrine and exocrine functions. Approximately how much of the mass of the pancreas is dedicated to exocrine function?
   A. 5%
   B. 25%
   C. 75%
   D. 95%

8. The primary hormone for stimulating secretion from the exocrine pancreas during a meal is
   A. cholecystokinin.
   B. gastrin.
   C. secretin.
   D. insulin.

TRUE/FALSE

Indicate whether the following statements are true (T) or false (F).

9. _____ Patients can have cholelithiasis but remain asymptomatic.

10. _____ Elevated serum amylase is the preferred laboratory test for the diagnosis of acute pancreatitis.

11. _____ Patients can develop cholecystitis without having gallstones present.

12. _____ The best diagnostic test for acute pancreatitis is an abdominal x-ray.

13. _____ Gallbladder disease is usually treated by removal of the gallbladder.

14. _____ In patients with chronic pancreatitis, therapeutic interventions include pain management.

FILL IN THE BLANKS

Fill in the blanks with the appropriate word or words.

15. Exiting the gallbladder, bile first travels through the _____ duct to join the _____ duct and form the _____ _____ duct.

16. Gallstone formation is enhanced by _____ of bile.

17. As an endocrine organ, the pancreas secretes _____, _____, and _____ into the bloodstream.

18. Most gallstones are made of _____.

19. Patients who are unable to tolerate cholecystectomy may be treated with _____ or _____.

20. In pancreatitis, digestive enzymes released into pancreatic tissues are activated and the resulting process is called _____.

38 Liver Diseases

TRUE/FALSE

Indicate whether the following questions are true (T) or false (F).

1. _____ The portal vein delivers venous blood to the liver from the entire gastrointestinal tract and the pancreas.

2. _____ Acute viral hepatitis can be more difficult to diagnose in the elderly.

3. _____ Portal hypertension results in decreased absorption of fat-soluble vitamins.

4. _____ Cystic fibrosis not only affects the lungs but can also cause forms of hepatitis and cirrhosis.

5. _____ Wilson disease is a hereditary disease due to a liver enzyme deficiency causing hepatic biliary obstruction.

6. _____ Hepatitis D virus infection requires a concurrent infection with the hepatitis A virus.

7. _____ One effect of hepatocellular failure is decreased production of albumin.

8. _____ An immature blood–brain barrier allows unconjugated bilirubin to cause kernicterus in premature neonates.

9. _____ Individuals who have alcohol-induced cirrhosis are not candidates for liver transplantation.

10. _____ Palmar erythema is a result of decreased production of clotting factors.

MULTIPLE CHOICE

Select the one best answer to each of the following questions.

11. Hepatocellular failure produces all of the following *except*
    A. jaundice.
    B. edema.
    C. bleeding tendencies.
    D. vitamin C deficiency.

12. An elevation in unconjugated bilirubin would be seen in all of the following *except*
    A. massive hemolysis.
    B. neonates.
    C. viral hepatitis.
    D. mechanical obstruction of the colon.

13. Impaired blood flow through the liver results in portal hypertension. This may produce
    A. osteomalacia.
    B. esophageal varices.
    C. impaired activation of vitamin D.
    D. hepatic coma.

14. The encephalopathy seen with liver failure is associated with the inability of the liver to
    A. conjugate bilirubin for excretion.
    B. synthesize albumin to maintain oncotic pressure.
    C. metabolize hormones, especially aldosterone and estrogen.
    D. convert ammonia to urea for excretion.

131

15. Acute renal failure secondary to liver failure (hepatorenal syndrome) is due to
    A. diminished blood flow to the kidneys.
    B. obstruction of the ureters as they exit the renal pelvis.
    C. accumulation of unmetabolized waste in the renal tubules.
    D. pressure on the renal arteries by ascitic fluid.

16. Hepatitis A
    A. is spread by contact with contaminated body fluids, such as blood or wound drainage.
    B. has an incubation period of up to 4 months.
    C. can be prevented through immunization.
    D. typically leaves the patient with permanently impaired liver function.

17. Hepatitis B and hepatitis C share a similar
    A. incubation period.
    B. prophylactic vaccine.
    C. incidence of progression to chronic liver disease.
    D. mode of transmission.

18. Chronic hepatitis, regardless of the specific disease, is characterized by
    A. continuing liver inflammation for 6 months or longer.
    B. a viral cause.
    C. progression to liver cancer or cirrhosis.
    D. diffuse scarring and fibrosis of the liver.

19. Though commonly called liver function tests (LFT), this laboratory evaluation actually measures
    A. enzymes indicative of acute liver damage.
    B. the amount of liver scarring.
    C. the amount of remaining functional liver tissue.
    D. toxin accumulation in the serum.

20. The underlying pathologic mechanism of hemochromatosis is
    A. excessive absorption of dietary iron.
    B. excessive accumulation of dietary copper.
    C. formation of excessive amounts of hemoglobin.
    D. formation of excessive amounts of activated vitamin D.

21. Children or adults consuming excessive amounts of acetaminophen are at risk for
    A. cirrhosis.
    B. liver necrosis.
    C. increased bleeding in the liver.
    D. impaired gastrointestinal functioning.

22. Cancer of the liver is
    A. a risk associated with hepatitis A.
    B. rarely associated with cirrhosis.
    C. usually due to metastasis from another site.
    D. most often managed by surgical resection.

23. Liver abscess
    A. may be due to infection with *Helicobacter pylori.*
    B. requires surgical intervention.
    C. should be considered in patients with fever and right upper quadrant pain.
    D. frequently recurs.

24. Trauma to the liver
    A. can result in significant blood loss into the abdomen.
    B. is only a concern with abdominal trauma.
    C. rarely requires surgical intervention.
    D. is accompanied by signs and symptoms of systemic infection.

25. All of the following are primary functions of the liver *except*
    A. clotting factor synthesis.
    B. erythropoietin synthesis.
    C. albumin synthesis.
    D. lipoprotein synthesis.

FILL IN THE BLANKS

Fill in the blanks with the appropriate word or words.

26. Patients with chronic alcoholic liver disease usually have a deficiency of vitamin _____ that impairs

    production of _____ _____.

27. Patients with liver failure commonly have generalized edema secondary to a reduction in synthesis of _____

    that reduces plasma _____ pressure.

28. Patients with liver disease that impairs excretion of bilirubin may exhibit a discoloration of the skin called

    _____.

29. Esophageal varices carry a high risk of _____ and may be treated with drugs to lower portal

    _____ _____.

30. The classic physical finding in patients with significant hepatic encephalopathy is a spastic movement of the hands

    called _____.

UNIT X: Case Studies

T.W. is a 52-year-old man who has developed cirrhosis secondary to repeated, prolonged exposure to alcohol. He has most recently been hospitalized because of an upper gastrointestinal bleed due to the rupture of esophageal varices

1. T.W.'s skin and the sclera of his eyes have a yellowish cast. The nurse knows that this jaundice is due to
   A. release of excessive amounts of iron from red blood cells.
   B. increased quantities of conjugated bilirubin.
   C. excessive contraction of the sphincter of Oddi.
   D. increased quantities of unconjugated bilirubin.

2. The development of esophageal varices in cirrhosis is related to
   A. hepatic fibrosis causing increased resistance to portal circulation.
   B. impairment of venous drainage from the thorax to the liver.
   C. increased vascular volume due to hepatorenal failure.
   D. pressure increases due to prolonged vomiting.

3. Early signs and symptoms characteristic of acute upper gastrointestinal hemorrhage due to esophageal varices include
   A. a rapid decrease in hematocrit.
   B. confusion, disorientation, and coma.
   C. hematemesis.
   D. abdominal distention.

133

4. Interventions that decrease portal hypertension responsible for esophageal varices include
   A. blood transfusions.
   B. endoscopic sclerosis.
   C. nitroglycerin and octreotide acetate.
   D. balloon tamponade.

5. Ruptured esophageal varices can produce profound hemorrhage. An additional pathologic feature of cirrhosis that contributes to hemorrhage is
   A. hypoalbuminemia.
   B. impaired production of clotting factors.
   C. altered production of lipoproteins.
   D. impaired glycogenesis and glycogenolysis.

C.D. comes to the clinic complaining of a long-lasting gastrointestinal flu. He tells the nurse that he became ill about a month after returning from a visit with friends in another state. Further investigation determines that one of C.D.'s friends has similar symptoms. Laboratory studies reveal a slight increase in aspartate aminotransferase (AST) levels, a total bilirubin of 1.5 mg/dl, and positive anti-hepatitis A virus IgM.

6. These laboratory tests are indicative of
   A. immunity to hepatitis A.
   B. previous infection with hepatitis A.
   C. active infection with hepatitis A.
   D. exposure to but no infection with hepatitis A.

7. Physical signs and symptoms of hepatitis include all of the following *except*
   A. anorexia.
   B. low-grade fever.
   C. acute left upper quadrant abdominal pain.
   D. nausea.

8. The most common means of contracting hepatitis A is
   A. poor personal hygiene.
   B. sexual intercourse.
   C. contaminated needles or blood transfusion.
   D. ingestion of contaminated food or water.

D.D. is a 43-year-old woman who comes into the emergency room complaining of acute abdominal pain. She states that the pain came on after dinner at an "all-you-can-eat" buffet and has been increasing steadily. The pain is located in her right upper quadrant and is "boring" into her back. She says she feels "gassy" and bloated.

9. The emergency department clinician suspects cholecystitis and orders
   A. a complete blood count.
   B. an abdominal x-ray.
   C. measurement of bilirubin levels.
   D. an abdominal ultrasound.

10. The cause of cholecystitis usually is
    A. a viral infection.
    B. hepatocellular failure.
    C. biliary obstruction by gallstones.
    D. biliary atresia.

11. The advantage of cholecystectomy over chemical dissolution and lithotripsy is
    A. decreased cost.
    B. no recurrence of the cholecystitis.
    C. less risk of diarrhea.
    D. fewer dietary alterations.

12. The principal complication of unmanaged cholecystitis is
    A. rupture of the gallbladder.
    B. sepsis.
    C. hemorrhage.
    D. inability to digest fats.

13. The most common point of biliary obstruction by cholelithiasis is
    A. the common bile duct.
    B. the cystic duct.
    C. the duodenal papilla.
    D. the sphincter of Oddi.

M.N. has rheumatoid arthritis and takes high doses of aspirin to control his pain and maintain function. He has had problems with gastritis from the aspirin, but it seemed to be relieved when he switched to enteric-coated aspirin and started taking it with food. Now, however, it seems to be worse. He came to the clinic complaining of increasing abdominal distress, and a gastric ulcer was diagnosed.

14. Aspirin and nonsteroidal antiinflammatory drugs (NSAIDs) are causative factors for the development of peptic ulcer disease (PUD) because they
    A. increase acid secretion.
    B. allow proliferation of *H. pylori.*
    C. damage the mucosal barrier.
    D. alter platelet aggregation.

15. Although by themselves they are not the cause of PUD, all of the following can contribute to the condition *except*
    A. smoking.
    B. caffeine.
    C. alcohol.
    D. estrogen.

16. M.N.'s therapy for his rheumatoid arthritis is changed. Another intervention that will contribute to the healing of his peptic ulcers is
    A. steroid administration.
    B. blocking or neutralizing of acid secretion.
    C. surgical removal of the ulcer.
    D. intravenous nutritional support.

17. Pepsin, a proteolytic enzyme found in the gastrointestinal tract, is converted from its precursor form, pepsinogen, in the presence of
    A. HCO_3^- secretions from the pancreas delivered to the duodenum.
    B. HCl secretions in the stomach.
    C. *H. pylori* bacteria, in residence in the epithelial wall.
    D. gastrin secretions in the stomach.

A.G. is a 32-year-old accountant who has been dealing with Crohn disease since her early twenties. She has had one bowel resection, which provided some improvement of symptoms for a few years. She comes to the clinic for a routine evaluation of her therapeutic regimen.

18. Crohn disease differs pathologically from ulcerative colitis in that ulcerative colitis
    A. affects only the mucosal layer of the bowel.
    B. involves the small and large bowel.
    C. produces a greater risk for malabsorption of nutrients.
    D. may progress to development of fistulas in adjacent organs.

19. Management of both Crohn disease and ulcerative colitis focuses on
    A. decreasing inflammation with drug therapy.
    B. reducing intake of foods that are high in fiber.
    C. limiting fluid intake during episodes of diarrhea.
    D. antibiotic therapy to eliminate the causative organisms.

20. Crohn disease and ulcerative colitis both
    A. typically develop in young adulthood.
    B. produce stool that is watery and filled with mucus and pus.
    C. have remissions, with full recovery of pathologic changes in the bowel.
    D. cause adhesions in the bowel.

39 Endocrine Physiology and Mechanisms of Hypothalamic-Pituitary Regulation

MATCHING

Match each definition on the left with its term on the right. Not all terms are defined.

1. _____ Prolonged exposure to high levels of a hormone can produce this response by the hormone receptors.

2. _____ Water-soluble hormones produce their effect by binding to cell membrane receptors that produce these within the cell.

3. _____ Chemical signals secreted by one cell that affect adjacent cells

4. _____ Hormones synthesized here travel via nerve axons to the posterior pituitary gland for release.

5. _____ Lipid-soluble hormones, like thyroid hormone, must be attached to these to be transported in the blood.

6. _____ Hormones that are lipid soluble and are derived from cholesterol are known as _____.

7. _____ Cortisol is an example of a hormone whose release varies over a 24-hour period, called a _____ pattern.

8. _____ This circulating thyroid hormone must be converted to its active form to be biologically active.

9. _____ Releasing hormones from the hypothalamus stimulate hormone secretion from the _____.

10. _____ The primary mechanism by which most hormone levels in the blood are controlled.

A. Steroids
B. Hypothalamus
C. Trophic hormone
D. Down-regulation
E. Paracrine
F. Up-regulation
G. Proteins
H. Autocrine
I. Second messengers
J. Lower
K. Anterior pituitary
L. Circadian
M. T_3
N. Positive feedback
O. T_4
P. Negative feedback

TRUE/FALSE

Indicate whether the following statements are true (T) or false (F).

11. _____ Release of the primary mineralocorticoid aldosterone is controlled by adrenocorticotropic hormone from the anterior pituitary gland.

12. _____ Norepinephrine, dopamine, and epinephrine are catecholamines that are water soluble.

13. _____ Hormone resistance can be identified when circulating levels of a hormone are normal or elevated but target organ function is deficient.

14. _____ Steroid hormones are easily excreted from the body and do not require metabolism.

15. _____ "Receptor specificity" means that the cells of a given tissue will respond only to hormones for which it has receptors.

16. _____ Receptor activation occurs when a hormone antagonist binds to the receptor.

137

17. _____ Phosphorylation–dephosphorylation is a common strategy for controlling enzyme activity in cells.

18. _____ Pharmacologic levels of hormones are higher than physiologic levels.

19. _____ Primary endocrine disease is differentiated from secondary endocrine disease because in primary disease the problem is with the target glands.

20. _____ More hormone is necessary to activate receptors when the receptors have a high affinity for the given hormone.

MULTIPLE CHOICE

Select the one best answer to each of the following questions.

21. Drugs that block dopamine activity are likely to increase the secretion of
    A. prolactin.
    B. thyroid-stimulating hormone.
    C. adrenocorticotropic hormone.
    D. growth hormone.

22. All of the following would be expected to raise blood glucose *except*
    A. growth hormone.
    B. cortisol.
    C. epinephrine.
    D. aldosterone.

23. Thyroid hormones are synthesized by the enzyme
    A. thyroid hydroxylase.
    B. thyroid peroxidase.
    C. thyroid synthase.
    D. colloid synthase.

24. The primary negative feedback for the release of corticotropin-releasing hormone (CRH) is
    A. insulin-like growth factor-1 (IGF-1).
    B. cortisol.
    C. glucose.
    D. aldosterone.

25. The portal vein transports releasing factors from the hypothalamus to the
    A. posterior pituitary.
    B. anterior pituitary.
    C. hypophyseal arteries.
    D. paraventricular area.

Chapter **39** Endocrine Physiology and Mechanisms of Hypothalamic-Pituitary Regulation

40 Disorders of Endocrine Function

FILL IN THE BLANKS

Fill in the blanks with the appropriate word or words.

1. An excess of growth hormone in adults is called _____, whereas in childhood it results in _____

   _____.

2. The primary intervention for syndrome of inappropriate antidiuretic hormone secretion (SIADH) is the restriction

   of _____ _____ intake.

3. Manifestations of hyperparathyroidism and hypoparathyroidism are related to excessive or insufficient amounts of

   serum _____.

4. Endocrine diseases characterized as hyporesponsive are clinically similar to hyposecretion of hormones but are

   due to _____ _____.

5. In primary hypothyroidism, the circulating level of thyroid-stimulating hormone (TSH) will be _____.

6. A unique feature of Graves disease is protrusion of the eyeballs, called _____.

7. The most common cause of hypoparathyroidism is _____ in the area where the glands are
   located.

8. A common cause of endocrine disorders, especially in women, is _____.

9. In adrenocortical deficiency, the most severe manifestations are related to inadequate quantities of the hormone

   _____.

10. A potentially lethal condition in which there is an acute elevation of circulating thyroid hormones is called

    _____ _____.

MULTIPLE CHOICE

Select the one best answer to each of the following questions.

11. Children with a deficiency in growth hormone may demonstrate which of the following manifestations?
    A. Early onset of puberty
    B. Bone overgrowth producing bony tumors
    C. Early loss of primary dentition
    D. Decreased height for chronologic age

12. Diabetes insipidus is characterized by
    A. hypernatremia.
    B. neurologic symptoms associated with swelling of brain cells.
    C. weight gain.
    D. increased urine-specific gravity.

13. Causes of acquired hypothyroidism include all of the following *except*
    A. goitrogenic foods.
    B. Hashimoto thyroiditis.
    C. thyroid gland agenesis.
    D. insufficient iodine intake.

14. Hypothyroidism manifestations include
    A. heat intolerance.
    B. moist, warm skin.
    C. nonpitting edema.
    D. insomnia.

15. In Graves disease
    A. circulating levels of thyroid hormones are decreased.
    B. an autoimmune process activates TSH receptors.
    C. the metabolic rate is slowed.
    D. the blood pressure drops significantly.

16. Congenital hypothyroidism that is not managed is a serious concern because of the risk for
    A. intellectual disability.
    B. respiratory distress.
    C. heart failure.
    D. seizures.

17. Parathyroid hormone normally exerts control over the serum calcium concentration by affecting all of the following *except*
    A. osteoclastic/osteoblastic activity.
    B. renal tubular reabsorption of calcium.
    C. gastrointestinal absorption of dietary calcium.
    D. synthesis of vitamin K.

18. A patient with hyperparathyroidism would be likely to present with
    A. elevated calcitonin levels.
    B. depressed deep tendon reflexes.
    C. numbness and tingling of the fingers or toes.
    D. Positive Chvostek sign.

19. A potentially life-threatening finding in hypoparathyroidism is
    A. laryngospasm.
    B. Trousseau sign.
    C. Chvostek sign.
    D. heart failure.

20. Cortisol, the body's primary glucocorticoid,
    A. is released from the anterior pituitary gland.
    B. increases glycogenesis.
    C. is a catabolic hormone.
    D. enhances the inflammatory response.

21. Findings associated with primary adrenal insufficiency/Addison disease include
    A. fluid retention.
    B. hypokalemia.
    C. hyperglycemia.
    D. hypovolemia.

22. Classic manifestations seen with Cushing syndrome include all of the following *except*
    A. bruising due to capillary fragility.
    B. hypertrophy of muscle tissue.
    C. increased susceptibility to infections.
    D. pathologic fractures.

23. Aldosterone promotes reabsorption of sodium and water, as well as excretion of potassium by the kidneys. What other hormone also produces these effects?
    A. Antidiuretic hormone
    B. Glucocorticoid hormone
    C. Thyroid hormone
    D. Parathyroid hormone

24. Pheochromocytoma is a rare, life-threatening disease characterized by
    A. intermittent severe hypertension.
    B. circulatory collapse from dehydration.
    C. respiratory arrest.
    D. total absence of a stress response.

25. Conn syndrome is characterized by
    A. secondary deficiency of cortisol.
    B. secondary deficiency of aldosterone.
    C. primary excess of cortisol.
    D. primary excess of aldosterone.

41 Diabetes Mellitus

TRUE/FALSE

Indicate whether the following statements are true (T) or false (F).

1. _____ Drug therapy for type 2 diabetes mellitus is the replacement of insulin, which is absent from the body.

2. _____ One of the classic clinical manifestations of diabetes mellitus is increased appetite, called polydipsia.

3. _____ Neurons do not require the presence of insulin to transport glucose.

4. _____ The primary source of energy for muscle tissue in the fasting or resting state is free fatty acids.

5. _____ Diabetic ketoacidosis and nonketotic hyperosmolar coma are most serious when they occur in the young.

6. _____ Risk factors for immune-mediated type 1 diabetes are genetic predisposition and environmental factors.

7. _____ Exercise requires an increase in insulin administration in patients with diabetes mellitus.

8. _____ Patients with type 2 diabetes mellitus may take both oral agents and injectable insulin.

9. _____ A significant risk factor for type 2 diabetes mellitus is obesity.

10. _____ Accumulation of autoantibodies against pancreatic β cells is associated with the progression of type 2 diabetes mellitus.

MULTIPLE CHOICE

Select the one best answer to each of the following questions.

11. All of the following hormones increase blood glucose levels *except*
    A. cortisol.
    B. oxytocin.
    C. growth hormone.
    D. norepinephrine.

12. Type 1 diabetes mellitus differs from type 2 in that
    A. the onset is usually in middle or later adulthood.
    B. it is associated with insulin resistance.
    C. it is the most common form of diabetes.
    D. there is an absolute deficiency of insulin production.

13. Ketoacidosis is uncommon in type 2 diabetes because
    A. dehydration is less severe.
    B. endogenous insulin prevents lipolysis and production of ketone bodies.
    C. metabolic acidosis does not occur.
    D. liver breakdown of stored glycogen does not produce fatty acids.

14. Women who develop gestational diabetes
    A. will probably remain diabetic following delivery of their babies.
    B. give birth to babies with low birth weights who are hyperglycemic.
    C. are primarily treated with any of the available oral agents.
    D. are likely to experience it with subsequent pregnancies.

15. Microvascular complications occurring with chronic hyperglycemia in diabetes mellitus include all of the following *except*
    A. peripheral arterial disease.
    B. retinopathy.
    C. nephropathy.
    D. neuropathy.

16. A sign of early diabetic nephropathy is
    A. anuria.
    B. glycosuria.
    C. hypertension.
    D. microalbuminuria.

17. Neuropathy of sensory nerves seen in diabetes mellitus is usually
    A. bilateral and may affect hands and feet.
    B. asymptomatic, painless.
    C. completely reversible with better diabetes management.
    D. controlled by medications that increase insulin production.

18. Diabetes mellitus is diagnosed when two fasting blood glucose samples are found to be greater than or equal to
    A. 100 mg/dL.
    B. 110 mg/dL.
    C. 126 mg/dL.
    D. 140 mg/dL.

19. Exercise for the patient with type 2 diabetes may result in
    A. improved renal function.
    B. decreased insulin resistance.
    C. decreased risk of eating disorder development.
    D. increased low-density lipid levels.

20. Signs or symptoms of hypoglycemia include all of the following *except*
    A. pallor.
    B. tremors.
    C. fever.
    D. altered consciousness.

21. Which of the following is *true* regarding complications of diabetes in children?
    A. Neuropathies are common and develop early in the disease.
    B. Diabetic ketoacidosis rarely occurs.
    C. Dehydration is a major concern when hyperglycemia is severe.
    D. Manifestations of hypoglycemia in very young children are identical to those seen in adults.

22. In the elderly population, complications of diabetes and aging increase the risk for the development of
    A. hyperglycemia.
    B. hypoglycemia.
    C. diabetic ketoacidosis.
    D. heart disease.

23. Measures of glycosylated hemoglobin, such as hemoglobin A_{1C} (HbA_{1C}), are used to monitor blood glucose control over the past
    A. 24 hours.
    B. week.
    C. month.
    D. 2 to 3 months.

24. Many diabetic patients are managed with basal-bolus insulin therapy, in which a long-acting insulin covers

_____ needs for insulin.
   A. acute.
   B. basal.
   C. nighttime.
   D. mealtime.

25. All of the following complications of diabetes mellitus result from excessive insulin exposure that contributes to macrovascular atherosclerosis *except*
   A. coronary artery disease.
   B. peripheral arterial disease.
   C. stroke.
   D. retinopathy.

42 Nutritional and Metabolic Disorders

FILL IN THE BLANKS

Fill in the blanks with the appropriate word or words.

1. _____ is the process of building body tissues and _____ is the process of breaking them down.

2. Two important factors that alter basal metabolic rate are _____ and _____.

3. When people are ill and in physiologic stress, the dominant metabolic process is _____.

4. Metabolic rates increase by _____ % for each degree Fahrenheit increase in body temperature.

5. The three organic nutrients are _____, _____, and _____.

6. A _____ nitrogen balance occurs when protein intake exceeds protein losses.

7. Two important hormonal regulators of appetite and food intake are _____ and _____.

8. Ketones are produced from incomplete metabolism of _____ _____.

MULTIPLE CHOICE

Select the one best answer to each of the following questions.

9. Biochemical tests indicative of either a poor intake of protein or protein use by the liver are
   A. low transferrin, albumin, and prealbumin levels.
   B. elevated blood urea nitrogen (BUN) and creatinine levels.
   C. decreased red blood cell and hemoglobin levels.
   D. increased hematocrit and white blood cell count.

10. Compared to fats, the use of glucose for adenosine triphosphate (ATP) production produces more
    A. energy.
    B. carbon dioxide.
    C. ATP.
    D. heat.

11. A significant complication that malnourished patients may develop when feeding is resumed is
    A. heart failure.
    B. infections.
    C. respiratory failure.
    D. muscle spasms.

12. Patients who are malnourished prior to surgery are at increased risk for
    A. impaired gastrointestinal motility.
    B. an increased basal metabolic rate.
    C. poor wound healing.
    D. muscle atrophy.

13. The basal metabolic rate
    A. increases with age.
    B. increases with the amount of lean muscle mass.
    C. is not significantly affected by ambient temperature.
    D. is not significantly affected by disease processes.

14. Normally, the primary nutrient source in the diet is
    A. glycogen.
    B. fats.
    C. carbohydrates.
    D. protein.

15. In a state of negative nitrogen balance,
    A. catabolism dominates.
    B. anabolism dominates.
    C. maximal growth occurs.
    D. carbohydrate metabolism predominates.

16. Most body tissues can efficiently metabolize and use fatty acids as an energy source as well as glucose *except*
    A. cardiac cells.
    B. brain cells.
    C. muscle cells.
    D. glandular cells.

17. One of the ways metabolism changes in the elderly is
    A. insulin sensitivity is decreased.
    B. serum lipid levels decline.
    C. insulin secretion is decreased.
    D. protein use in gluconeogenesis increases.

18. Important hormonal regulators of nutrient metabolism include all of the following *except*
    A. cortisol.
    B. growth hormone.
    C. glucagon.
    D. parathyroid hormone.

19. Classic features of metabolic syndrome include all of the following *except*
    A. increased abdominal circumference.
    B. elevated blood pressure.
    C. low high-density lipoprotein (HDL) cholesterol.
    D. reduced secretion of insulin.

TRUE/FALSE

Indicate whether the following statements are true (T) or false (F).

20. _____ Dietary fats provide 9 kilocalories per gram.

21. _____ On a per-gram basis, carbohydrates provide more kilocalories than protein.

22. _____ Carbohydrates can be converted to fats in cells that have carbohydrate excess.

23. _____ Obesity is defined as a body mass index (BMI) of more than 30 kg/m^2.

24. _____ Ketones are a significant source of energy for cells during periods of starvation.

25. _____ The primary source of energy during prolonged fasting is body fat.

UNIT XI: Case Studies

Eight-year-old W.E. has been brought to the doctor's office by his parents. Over the past few days, he has been weak, complaining of being very thirsty and hungry. They have noticed he urinates more frequently. Laboratory tests in combination with this history confirm the diagnosis of type 1 diabetes mellitus.

1. The polyuria associated with diabetes is due to
   A. the polydipsia.
   B. the osmotic effects of glycosuria.
   C. increased protein catabolism.
   D. the loss of electrolytes.

2. Excessive ketone production may produce what laboratory finding?
   A. Increased partial pressure of carbon dioxide
   B. Decreased hematocrit
   C. Decreased pH
   D. Increased BUN level

3. The rapid, deep respirations associated with ketoacidosis (Kussmaul respirations) are the result of the body's attempt to
   A. compensate for metabolic acidosis.
   B. combat hypoxemia.
   C. increase the partial pressure of oxygen.
   D. improve the level of consciousness.

4. Because W.E. has type 1 diabetes, insulin therapy will be required. At his age, W.E. can be taught to monitor his blood sugar and administer his own insulin injections with supervision. All of the following statements regarding pediatric considerations in the administration of insulin and monitoring of blood glucose levels are true *except*
   A. adequate treatment is essential to ensure normal growth and maturation.
   B. insulin injections should be given only in the abdomen.
   C. an intensive regimen of at least three injections per day helps to avoid chronic complications.
   D. if doses are very small, a diluent may be needed to ensure adequate drug delivery.

5. The best laboratory test to monitor how well W.E.'s blood sugar levels are being managed over time is
   A. testing for glucose in the urine.
   B. the fasting blood glucose level.
   C. spot checking the blood glucose level.
   D. the glycosylated hemoglobin (HbA_{1C}) test.

N.M., a 45-year-old woman, was diagnosed with hypothyroidism 10 years ago. Her condition has been effectively managed with thyroid replacement therapy.

6. The most likely cause of N.M.'s hypothyroidism would be a history of
   A. cretinism.
   B. thyroid dysgenesis.
   C. Hashimoto thyroiditis.
   D. Graves disease.

7. Laboratory results that would indicate a primary cause of hypothyroidism would be decreased thyroxine (T4) and
   A. increased thyroid-stimulating hormone (TSH).
   B. decreased TSH.
   C. increased thyrotropin-releasing hormone (TRH).
   D. decreased TRH.

8. When N.M. came to see her doctor 10 years ago, which of the following complaints would have been associated with hypothyroidism?
   A. Diarrhea
   B. Jaundice
   C. Weight loss
   D. Menstrual irregularity

A type 2 diabetic for more than 25 years, C.T. is now nearly 80 years old. His primary health care problems are related to the chronic complications of diabetes.

9. The primary risk factor for type 2 diabetes is
   A. ethnicity.
   B. obesity.
   C. autoimmune disease.
   D. heredity.

10. In type 2 diabetes, the pathologic process involves
    A. decreased glucagon secretion.
    B. an absolute deficiency of insulin.
    C. decreased tissue sensitivity to insulin.
    D. anti-insulin antibody formation.

11. Physiologic changes associated with his age, coupled with pathophysiologic alterations related to his diabetes, increase C.T.'s risk for
    A. hemorrhagic stroke.
    B. osteoporosis.
    C. myocardial infarction.
    D. presbyopia.

12. A condition that contributes to the development of diabetic nephropathy is
    A. hypertension.
    B. autonomic neuropathy.
    C. renal calculi.
    D. prostate cancer.

13. Which of the following observations is likely associated with a chronic complication of C.T.'s diabetes?
    A. C.T. wears a hearing aid.
    B. C.T. wears glasses to read.
    C. C.T. has partial dentures.
    D. C.T. has a below-the-knee amputation.

P.B. is a 43-year-old electrical engineer. He arrives in the emergency department by ambulance, where the paramedics and his wife report a sudden onset of nausea, vomiting, and diarrhea. His blood pressure is very low, and laboratory findings include low blood sugar and profoundly increased serum potassium.

14. This scenario suggests what endocrine emergency?
    A. Thyroid storm
    B. Addisonian crisis
    C. Pheochromocytoma
    D. Diabetic ketoacidosis

15. Appropriate treatment of P.B. requires
    A. intravenous thyroid hormone replacement.
    B. intravenous insulin administration.
    C. immediate surgery to remove a tumor.
    D. intravenous administration of glucocorticoid.

16. Once he has been treated and routine medications have been established, P.B. should be urged to

    avoid _____ to decrease the likelihood of recurrence of an emergency.
    A. foods high in carbohydrates
    B. emotional and physical stressors
    C. overdosage of his medication
    D. excessive fluid intake

S.Z. underwent kidney transplantation 3 years ago and has been taking steroids to suppress the immune response and reduce the risk of organ rejection. This medication has produced Cushing syndrome.

17. Although she is only 38 years old, S.Z.'s Cushing syndrome places her at increased risk for what condition that is normally found in people much older than she?
    A. Heart disease
    B. Renal insufficiency
    C. Osteoporosis
    D. Menopause

18. S.Z.'s blood pressure is carefully monitored because steroids can cause hypertension due to their propensity to cause
    A. increased contractility of the heart.
    B. atherosclerosis.
    C. sodium and water retention.
    D. increased heart rate.

19. Ecchymoses found on S.Z.'s legs after minor injuries are related to which of the following effects of long-term glucocorticoid administration?
    A. Protein catabolism causing capillary fragility
    B. Increased platelet aggregation
    C. Decreased glucose use
    D. Increased glycogenolysis

20. S.Z.'s routine laboratory testing reflects what common finding associated with increased cortisol levels?
    A. Decreased hemoglobin
    B. Increased serum potassium
    C. Decreased BUN levels
    D. Increased blood sugar

43 Structure and Function of the Nervous System

MATCHING

1. *Match each of the following anatomic terms with the appropriate letter in the figure.*

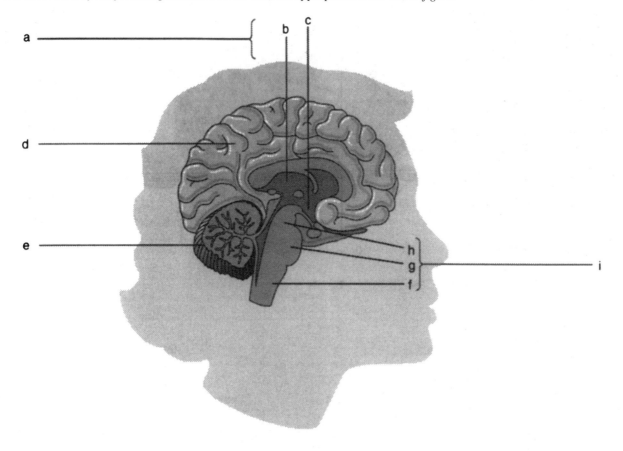

_____ Hypothalamus

_____ Medulla oblongata

_____ Brainstem

_____ Cerebrum

_____ Midbrain

_____ Thalamus

_____ Cerebellum

_____ Diencephalon

_____ Pons

2. *Match each of the following anatomic terms with the appropriate letter in the figure.*

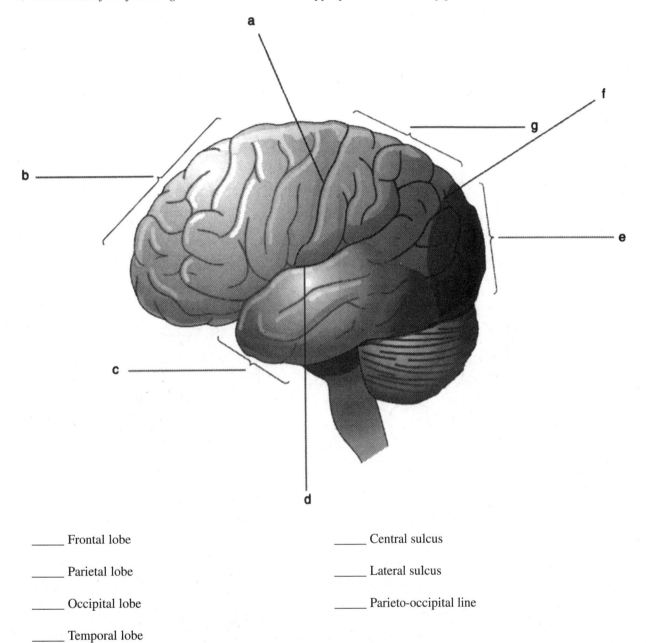

_____ Frontal lobe   _____ Central sulcus

_____ Parietal lobe   _____ Lateral sulcus

_____ Occipital lobe   _____ Parieto-occipital line

_____ Temporal lobe

     Chapter **43 Structure and Function of the Nervous System**

3. *Match each of the following anatomic terms with the appropriate letter in the figure.*

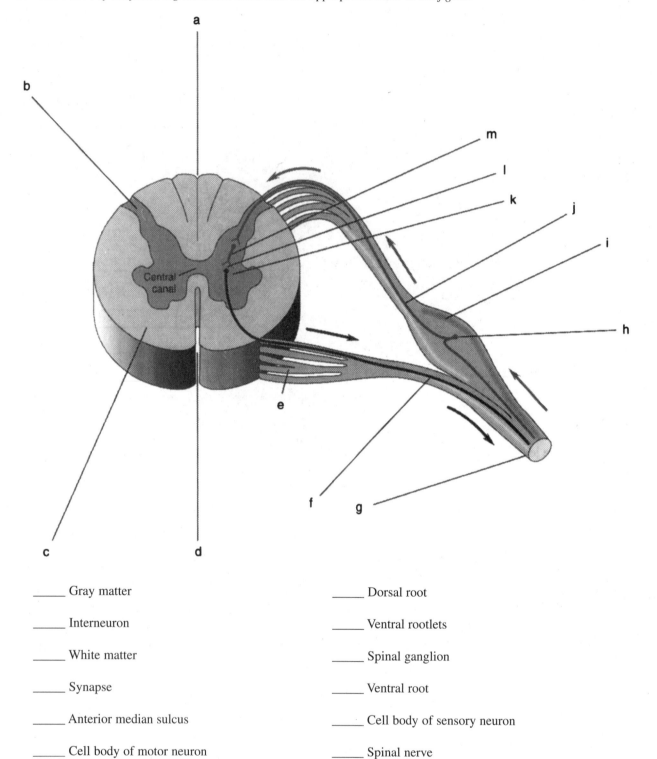

_____ Gray matter

_____ Interneuron

_____ White matter

_____ Synapse

_____ Anterior median sulcus

_____ Cell body of motor neuron

_____ Posterior median sulcus

_____ Dorsal root

_____ Ventral rootlets

_____ Spinal ganglion

_____ Ventral root

_____ Cell body of sensory neuron

_____ Spinal nerve

4. *Match each of the following anatomic terms with the appropriate letter in the figure.*

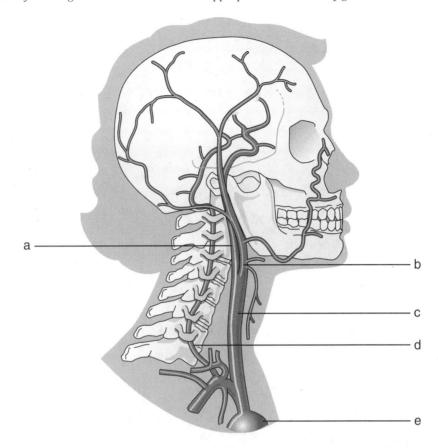

_____ Vertebral artery

_____ Internal carotid artery

_____ Aortic arch

_____ External carotid artery

_____ Common carotid artery

Chapter **43 Structure and Function of the Nervous System**

5. *Match each of the following anatomic terms with the appropriate letter in the figure.*

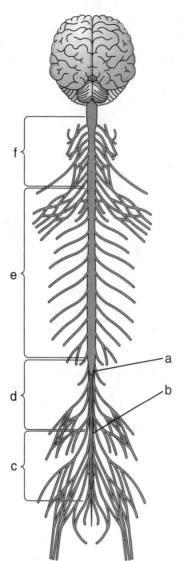

_____ Lumbar segments

_____ Cauda equina

_____ Cervical segments

_____ Sacral segments

_____ Conus medullaris

_____ Thoracic segments

Chapter **43 Structure and Function of the Nervous System**

Match each of the receptors on the left with the correct receptor class on the right. Answers may be used more than once.

6. _____ 5-Hydroxytryptamine 3 (5-HT$_3$)

7. _____ α-, β-Adrenergic

8. _____ 5-HT$_1$, 5-HT$_2$

9. _____ Gamma-aminobutyric acid type A (GABA$_A$)

10. _____ Nicotinic acetylcholine

11. _____ Muscarinic acetylcholine

A. Metabotropic receptor
B. Ionotropic receptor

Match each of the channel responses on the left with the type of postsynaptic potential it generates on the right. Answers may be used more than once.

12. _____ Na$^+$ channel opening

13. _____ K$^+$ channel opening

14. _____ Ca^{2+} channel opening

15. _____ Cl$^-$ channel opening

A. Inhibitory postsynaptic potential
B. Excitatory postsynaptic potential

Match each of the neural structures on the left with its description or function on the right. Answers may be used once or not at all.

16. _____ Anterolateral (spinothalamic) tract

17. _____ Corticospinal tracts

18. _____ Dorsal column, medial lemniscal tracts

19. _____ Occipital lobe

20. _____ Parietal lobe

21. _____ Frontal lobe

22. _____ Temporal lobe

23. _____ Thalamus

24. _____ Microglia

25. _____ Choroid ependymal cells

26. _____ Astrocytes

27. _____ Basal ganglia

28. _____ Extrapyramidal tracts

A. Transmit axial motor control
B. Site of primary auditory cortex
C. Cells that produce cerebrospinal fluid (CSF)
D. Transmit fine voluntary motor control
E. Transmit fine touch, proprioception
F. Site of primary motor cortex
G. Site of primary somatosensory cortex
H. Transmit pain, itch, temperature
I. Site of primary visual cortex
J. Structures involved in emotion
K. Relay center of the brain
L. Help maintain blood–brain barrier
M. Macrophages of the central nervous system (CNS)
N. Structures that plan motor programs
O. Parasympathetic tract

TRUE/FALSE

Indicate whether the following statements are true (T) or false (F).

29. _____ The peripheral nervous system includes 31 pairs of spinal nerves and 12 pairs of cranial nerves.

30. _____ The outermost layer of the brain meninges is the arachnoid.

31. _____ The epidural space lies between the pia mater and the dura mater.

32. _____ Cerebrospinal fluid (CSF) circulates in the subarachnoid space.

33. _____ The sympathetic nerves originate in spinal cord segments T1 to L2.

34. _____ There are two sets of basal ganglia, one in each cerebral hemisphere.

Chapter **43** **Structure and Function of the Nervous System**

35. _____ The pia mater is adherent to the surface of the brain.

36. _____ The primary motor cortex is located in the parietal lobe.

37. _____ The signal-receiving area of the neuron is the axon.

38. _____ Conduction of action potentials is faster in larger-diameter neurons.

39. _____ Glutamate functions as an inhibitory neurotransmitter in the CNS.

40. _____ Excitatory postsynaptic potential results from the opening of potassium and chloride channels in the post-synaptic neuron.

41. _____ Oligodendroglial cells form myelin in the CNS, whereas Schwann cells form myelin in the peripheral nervous system.

42. _____ The primary means of clearing amine neurotransmitters from the synapse is by active reuptake into pre-synaptic neurons.

43. _____ The thalamus acts as a processor and relay center for both afferent and efferent signals between the cerebral cortex and the brainstem.

MULTIPLE CHOICE

Select the one best answer to each of the following questions.

44. Neurons principally communicate through
    A. action potentials.
    B. chemical synapses.
    C. electrical signals.
    D. gap junctions.

45. The neurotransmitter class of amines includes all of the following neurotransmitters *except*
    A. serotonin.
    B. norepinephrine.
    C. dopamine.
    D. acetylcholine.

46. Which of the following neurotransmitters is always inhibitory?
    A. Acetylcholine
    B. Dopamine
    C. GABA
    D. Norepinephrine

47. Inhibitory neurotransmitters produce inhibitory postsynaptic potentials by
    A. opening voltage-gated sodium channels.
    B. opening ligand-gated sodium channels.
    C. opening chloride or potassium channels.
    D. opening calcium channels.

48. Touch receptors and proprioceptors on the left side of the body
    A. project to the left somatosensory cortex.
    B. travel up the ipsilateral spinal cord in the dorsal column.
    C. travel up the contralateral spinal cord in the anterolateral column.
    D. cross at the level of entry to the cord and synapse on interneurons.

49. The primary somatosensory and primary motor cortices are
    A. somatotopically organized.
    B. located in the frontal lobe.
    C. under control of the basal ganglia.
    D. organized into three structural layers.

156

50. Motor neurons from the corticospinal tract decussate at the
    A. corpus callosum.
    B. spinal cord.
    C. medullary pyramids.
    D. internal capsule.

51. The principal role of the cerebellum in motor activity is to
    A. plan the motor program.
    B. activate the α motor neurons in the spinal cord.
    C. improve the match between the intended movement and the actual movement.
    D. provide the motivational force for initiating movement.

52. Eliciting deep tendon reflexes is a test of
    A. spinal cord function.
    B. the monosynaptic stretch reflex.
    C. the Golgi tendon organ.
    D. the flexion withdrawal reflex.

53. Rapid eye movement (REM) sleep is associated with
    A. slow electroencephalographic waves.
    B. dream states.
    C. the most restful type of sleep.
    D. increased muscle tone and motor activity during sleep.

FILL IN THE BLANKS

Fill in the blanks with the appropriate word or words.

54. Action potentials are usually generated at the initial segment of a neuron because the threshold is _____

    due to an increased density of _____ _____ _____.

55. The *N*-methyl-D-aspartate (NMDA) receptor is a _____ ion channel that binds to the neurotransmitter

    _____, but will not open unless the membrane is partially depolarized, because in the polarized state a

    _____ ion normally blocks the channel.

56. Glial cells perform many supportive functions in the nervous system, but they do not have voltage-gated ion channels

    and therefore cannot _____ _____ _____.

57. The six general classes of neurotransmitters are

    1. _____

    2. _____

    3. _____

    4. _____

    5. _____

    6. _____

58. Low serum calcium ion levels in the extracellular fluid reduce neuronal _____ and increase neuromuscular

    _____.

59. The visual cortex is located in the _____ lobe.

60. Emotional responses are anatomically associated with the _____ system in the brain.

Chapter **43 Structure and Function of the Nervous System**

44 Acute Disorders of Brain Function

FILL IN THE BLANKS

Fill in the blanks with the appropriate word or words.

1. Symptoms suggestive of transient ischemic attack (TIA) are expected to resolve completely within _____ hours after onset.

2. Polar primary injury in traumatic brain injury results in damage to opposite sides of the brain due to _____ movement within the rigid skull.

3. Damage to the Broca area of the brain, most commonly associated with a left-sided stroke, will result in a patient's having difficulty with _____.

4. Although rarely diagnosed in the pediatric population, arteriovenous malformations are vascular abnormalities believed to be present at _____.

5. An etiologic difference between meningitis and encephalitis is that meningitis is usually due to a _____ infection, whereas encephalitis is typically due to a _____ infection.

6. The most significant risk for cerebral aneurysm rupture is _____.

7. _____ stroke has both higher mortality rates and higher morbidity rates than _____ stroke.

8. Many of the brain's intracellular enzyme systems are affected by _____ ions, which accumulate excessively following acute injury and are a significant factor in brain cell damage.

9. The damage produced by the infusion of inflammatory cells and development of oxygen-free radicals into an area previously ischemic is called _____ _____.

10. _____ edema develops when cell membrane pumps are unable to prevent an increase in cellular volume, and _____ edema occurs with changes within blood vessels that increase interstitial volume.

MULTIPLE CHOICE

Select the one best answer to each of the following questions.

11. A critical event in determining whether an injured neuronal cell will die or recover is the
    A. rate of action potential conduction.
    B. degree of intracellular calcium overload.
    C. degree of hypoglycemia.
    D. dysfunction of Na^+-K^+ pumps.

12. Hyperventilation to reduce Pa_{CO_2} is likely to produce
    A. cerebral vasoconstriction.
    B. cerebral hyperoxygenation.
    C. increased cerebral perfusion.
    D. cerebral vasodilation.

158

13. The brain's normal response to an increase in metabolism or a decrease in arterial perfusion pressure is to
    A. decrease metabolism.
    B. decrease blood flow.
    C. increase glucose use.
    D. vasodilate.

14. A decrease in the size of the cerebral ventricles on computed tomography (CT) scan is indicative of
    A. hydrocephalus.
    B. increased intracranial pressure (ICP).
    C. subarachnoid hemorrhage.
    D. Alzheimer disease.

15. Normal ICP ranges from
    A. 0 to 15 mm Hg.
    B. 5 to 25 mm Hg.
    C. 10 to 50 mm Hg.
    D. 25 to 50 mm Hg.

16. The earliest indicator of compromised neurologic functioning is usually
    A. an altered pupil light reflex.
    B. a change in level of consciousness.
    C. depressed motor responses.
    D. failure to follow commands.

17. The Glasgow Coma Scale has three measures of coma that include all of the following *except* the
    A. eye opening response.
    B. pupillary response.
    C. verbal response.
    D. motor response.

18. Which of the following responses represents the worst neurologic status?
    A. Opens eyes to pain
    B. Withdraws an extremity from pain
    C. Wiggles the toes to command
    D. Assumes a decorticate posture

19. Most severe head injuries are incurred in
    A. falls.
    B. motor vehicle accidents.
    C. diving accidents.
    D. sports accidents.

20. Characteristics of epidural hematoma include
    A. a slow progression of bleeding and increased ICP.
    B. venous bleeding from bridging veins.
    C. a lucid interval immediately after injury, followed by a rapid decline in the level of consciousness.
    D. extensive primary injury to neuronal structures.

21. The patient most at risk for central nervous system (CNS) infection following trauma is one with
    A. multiple scalp lacerations and abrasions after a fall.
    B. a closed head injury after falling off a trampoline.
    C. a basal skull fracture after falling off a ladder.
    D. a laceration of the face and scalp after being hit with a rusty pipe.

159

22. The most common cause of stroke is
    A. embolism.
    B. hemorrhage.
    C. thrombosis.
    D. trauma.

23. Patients who experience transient ischemic attacks (TIAs) are at increased risk for
    A. embolic stroke.
    B. hemorrhagic stroke.
    C. thrombotic stroke.
    D. hypertensive stroke.

24. Which of the following is a significant risk factor for the development of embolic stroke?
    A. Atrial fibrillation
    B. Deep vein thrombosis
    C. Hypertension
    D. Atherosclerosis

25. Typical manifestations of a stroke on the right side of the brain include
    A. significant aphasia.
    B. weakness on the right side of the body.
    C. loss of vision in the left visual field.
    D. a positive Babinski sign on the right foot.

26. Subarachnoid hemorrhage is most commonly a consequence of
    A. head trauma.
    B. cerebral aneurysm rupture.
    C. atherosclerotic plaque rupture.
    D. a bleeding disorder.

27. A patient with a headache, stiff neck, fever, and elevated cerebrospinal fluid (CSF) white blood cell count most likely has
    A. encephalitis.
    B. meningitis.
    C. cerebral abscess.
    D. neuralgia.

28. The pupil response to light tests the functioning of cranial nerves
    A. I and II.
    B. II and III.
    C. III and IV.
    D. III and VI.

29. The excitatory amino acid _____ can have neurotoxic effects on neurons when it is excessive in the synapse after injury.
    A. glutamate
    B. gamma-aminobutyric acid (GABA)
    C. glycine
    D. lysine

30. A person with head trauma who experiences 15 seconds of loss of consciousness following the injury has a grade

    _____ concussion.
    A. 0
    B. I
    C. II
    D. III

45 Chronic Disorders of Neurologic Function

MULTIPLE CHOICE

Select the one best answer to each of the following questions.

1. Clinical manifestations of a seizure depend on all of the following *except* the
   A. part of the brain involved.
   B. age of the patient.
   C. epileptogenic focus.
   D. areas of the brain recruited.

2. Seizures are classified as general when they
   A. are recurrent.
   B. involve both hemispheres of the brain.
   C. produce the same changes on electroencephalogram (EEG).
   D. are preceded by an aura.

3. Status epilepticus is of greatest concern in the patient with tonic–clonic seizures because
   A. patients are most likely to be injured.
   B. it often occurs at night.
   C. there is no satisfactory intervention.
   D. respiration ceases until the end of the clonic phase.

4. A patient with dementia and brain atrophy on computed tomography scanning or magnetic resonance imaging is likely to have
   A. a brain tumor.
   B. a brain infarction.
   C. vascular dementia.
   D. Alzheimer-type dementia.

5. Alzheimer disease is associated with excessive _____ in the brain.
   A. dendritic fibrils
   B. neurotransmitter release
   C. synaptic transmissions
   D. amyloid plaques

6. Parkinson disease is associated with a deficiency of basal ganglia
   A. norepinephrine.
   B. dopamine.
   C. gamma-aminobutyric acid (GABA).
   D. acetylcholine.

7. All of the following medications might be appropriate to manage the symptoms of Parkinson disease *except*
   A. a dopamine precursor (L-dopa).
   B. acetylcholine antagonists.
   C. monoamine oxidase inhibitors.
   D. a dopamine-receptor antagonist.

161

8. Clinical manifestations of cerebellar disorders include all of the following *except*
   A. ataxia.
   B. intention tremor.
   C. clumsiness.
   D. paralysis.

9. A patient who experiences lower extremity weakness but has normal sensation is likely to have
   A. multiple sclerosis.
   B. Guillain-Barré syndrome.
   C. spinal shock.
   D. peripheral neuropathy.

10. A congenital anomaly of the spinal cord in which the spinal nerves and meninges protrude from the back is termed
    A. spina bifida occulta.
    B. meningocele.
    C. myelomeningocele.
    D. spina bifida apparenta.

11. The major risk factors for the development of Alzheimer disease are age and
    A. alcoholism.
    B. stroke.
    C. family history.
    D. Parkinson disease.

12. Cerebral palsy is primarily a disorder of
    A. cognitive function.
    B. motor function.
    C. dopamine receptors.
    D. medullary neurons.

13. All of the following statements regarding amyotrophic lateral sclerosis (ALS) are true *except*
    A. cognitive function is impaired.
    B. it affects lower motor neurons.
    C. it is a progressive degenerative disease.
    D. it affects upper motor neurons.

14. Both multiple sclerosis and Guillain-Barré syndrome are demyelinating diseases that differ in that Guillain-Barré syndrome involves the
    A. upper motor neurons.
    B. lower motor neurons.
    C. autonomic neurons.
    D. central nervous system.

15. Bell palsy is most likely from
    A. autoimmune activation.
    B. bacterial infection.
    C. malignant transformation.
    D. viral infection.

FILL IN THE BLANKS

Fill in the blanks with the appropriate word or words.

16. Myasthenia gravis is a "grave weakness" that worsens with activity and is due to insufficient activity of _____ in the myoneural synapse.

17. Intention tremor is indicative of dysfunction of the _____, whereas a tremor at rest is indicative of _____

    _____.

18. Autonomic dysreflexia is a complication of spinal cord injury that occurs when the _____ nervous system is inappropriately activated below the level of injury, resulting in dangerously elevated _____ _____.

19. In normal-pressure hydrocephalus, the _____ of cerebrospinal fluid (CSF) increases without a change in intracranial pressure because there is a _____ in brain tissue volume.

20. The demyelination of nerve axons in multiple sclerosis is due to the inappropriate activation of the _____ system.

TRUE/FALSE

Indicate whether the following statements are true (T) or false (F).

21. _____ Dopamine agonist drugs are likely to cause or exacerbate Parkinson symptoms.

22. _____ A patient with pain in the C7 dermatome of the right arm and hand would be diagnosed with a peripheral neuropathy.

23. _____ A patient with a complete spinal cord injury at C4 is likely to have difficulty breathing and clearing the airways.

24. _____ The period of spinal shock that immediately follows complete spinal cord injury is characterized by spasticity and hyperreflexia.

25. _____ Neurofibrillary tangles and beta-amyloid plaques are the characteristic brain lesions of Alzheimer disease.

46 Alterations in Special Sensory Function

MATCHING

1. Match each of the following anatomic terms with the appropriate letter in the figure.

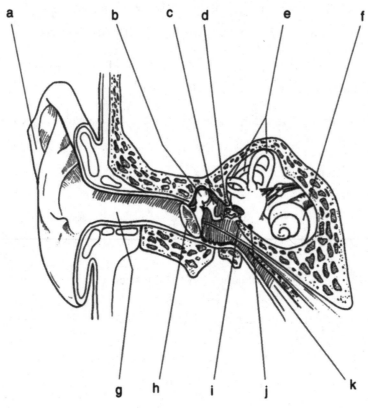

_____ Auricle

_____ Ear canal

_____ Incus

_____ Malleus

_____ Stapes

_____ Cochlea

_____ Semicircular canals

_____ Eustachian tube

_____ Round window

_____ Oval window

_____ Tympanic membrane

2. Match each of the following anatomic terms with the appropriate letter in the figure.

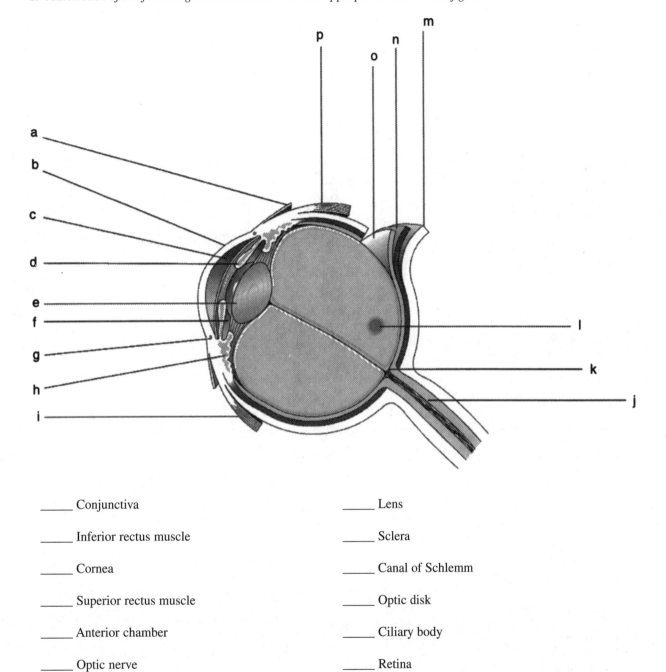

_____ Conjunctiva

_____ Inferior rectus muscle

_____ Cornea

_____ Superior rectus muscle

_____ Anterior chamber

_____ Optic nerve

_____ Iris

_____ Macula

_____ Lens

_____ Sclera

_____ Canal of Schlemm

_____ Optic disk

_____ Ciliary body

_____ Retina

_____ Posterior chamber

_____ Choroid

Chapter **46 Alterations in Special Sensory Function**

Select the one best answer to each of the following questions.

3. Movement of the tympanic membrane in the ear initiates movement of the malleolus, whereas movement of the oval window causes movement of the
   A. stapes.
   B. incus.
   C. perilymph.
   D. hair cells.

4. In the eye, the effect of sympathetic nervous system stimulation is
   A. contraction of ciliary muscle fibers.
   B. pupillary dilation.
   C. increased sensitivity of retinal rods.
   D. loss of the consensual response.

5. Vertigo commonly occurs with the auditory disorder called
   A. presbycusis.
   B. otitis media.
   C. Meniere disease.
   D. otosclerosis.

6. Conductive hearing disorders are a result of pathologic lesions of the
   A. external and/or middle ear.
   B. inner ear.
   C. hair cells.
   D. vestibulocochlear nerve.

7. Ossification of the bones of the middle ear is an example of
   A. presbycusis.
   B. a conductive abnormality.
   C. a sensorineural abnormality.
   D. otitis.

8. Otitis media commonly occurs in children with
   A. otitis externa.
   B. excessive exposure to loud noise.
   C. a foreign body in the ear canal.
   D. eustachian tube dysfunction.

9. An irregular curvature of the cornea or lens results in
   A. myopia.
   B. hyperopia.
   C. amblyopia.
   D. astigmatism.

10. Patients with diabetes mellitus are at particularly high risk and should be routinely evaluated for
    A. presbyopia.
    B. vascular retinopathy.
    C. retinal holes and tears.
    D. glaucoma.

11. Which of the following is characteristic of closed-angle glaucoma but not of open-angle glaucoma?
    A. Increased intraocular pressure
    B. Impaired visual acuity
    C. Acute eye pain
    D. Potential for blindness if untreated

12. An individual who experiences a change in olfactory sensation in the absence of an obvious etiologic factor, such as cold, inflammation, or smoke inhalation, should be evaluated for
    A. nasal polyps.
    B. a brain tumor.
    C. a nasal foreign body.
    D. deviation of the nasal septum.

FILL IN THE BLANKS

Fill in the blanks with the appropriate word or words.

13. Most ototoxic drugs affect _____ cells of the _____.

14. The two diseases most frequently associated with the development of retinopathy are _____ and _____ _____.

15. _____ detachment of the retina is most common in those over the age of 50 years.

16. The most common cause of decreased vision in children is _____.

17. When the eye is elongated and the resulting image focuses in front of the retina, the condition is called _____; a shorter eye resulting in the image focusing behind the retina is called _____; and a loss of the ability to accommodate is called _____.

18. The surgical removal of the lens of the eye is the treatment for a _____.

19. The leading cause of irreversible loss of vision in elderly persons is _____ _____ _____.

20. An important safety intervention for those with a diminished sense of smell is the installation of _____ _____.

TRUE/FALSE

Indicate whether the following statements are true (T) or false (F).

21. _____ Cranial nerve VIII transmits auditory and vestibular sensations to the brain.

22. _____ Otosclerosis is a term that refers to fusion or stiffness of bones in the middle ear.

23. _____ Buzzing or ringing in the ears is called presbycusis.

24. _____ Noise-induced sensorineural hearing loss is irreversible.

25. _____ Cataracts are found only in elderly persons.

47 Pain

MATCHING

Match each structure on the right with its description or function on the left. Answers may be used once or not at all.

1. _____ Free nerve endings for pain

2. _____ Myelinated A delta fibers

3. _____ Pain due to nerve damage

4. _____ Implicated in chronic pain syndromes

5. _____ Involved in pain modulation

6. _____ Location of pain nerve cell bodies

7. _____ Unmyelinated C fibers

8. _____ Level of stimulation necessary to perceive pain

A. Transmit slow pain sensation
B. Neuropathic pain
C. Pain threshold
D. Nociceptors
E. Transmit fast pain sensation
F. Anterior root
G. Acetylcholine
H. Pain tolerance
I. Dorsal root
J. Glutamate
K. Substance P
L. Gate control theory

MULTIPLE CHOICE

Select the one best answer to each of the following questions.

9. The perception of pain can be modulated by endogenous opioids called
   A. serotonins.
   B. endorphins and enkephalins.
   C. morphines.
   D. catecholamines.

10. The findings of increased blood pressure, pulse, and respiration in a patient are characteristic of pain that is
    A. chronic.
    B. acute.
    C. referred.
    D. psychogenic.

11. Painful stimulation of neurons in visceral structures is often perceived in another area because it is referred to
    A. the overlying skin.
    B. the spinal cord or nerve roots.
    C. structures from the same dermatome.
    D. phantom structures.

12. Cancer pain differs from other types of chronic pain in that it often
    A. is referred pain.
    B. is due to an excessive amount of gamma-aminobutyric acid (GABA).
    C. has an association with excess sympathetic innervation.
    D. has an identifiable cause.

13. Neuropathic pain is thought to result from
    A. altered central nervous system processing of nociceptive input.
    B. insufficient oxygen to nerve cells.
    C. changes in impulse modulation.
    D. injury along a dermatome.

168

14. Important chemical mediators of pain include all of the following *except*
    A. histamine.
    B. prostaglandins.
    C. thyroid hormone.
    D. lactate.

15. A significant aspect of pain in both elderly and very young persons is
    A. nociceptors are less sensitive.
    B. both groups respond best to interventions modulating pain transmission.
    C. pain perception is decreased.
    D. both groups are often undertreated.

16. Nociceptors are found in all of the following locations *except*
    A. brain tissue.
    B. viscera.
    C. muscle.
    D. connective tissue.

FILL IN THE BLANKS

Fill in the blanks with the appropriate word or words.

17. The _____ drugs interfere with pain perception in the brain, whereas nociceptor activation is altered peripherally by _____ _____ and _____ _____, and the application of _____ and _____.

18. Poorly localized pain that is perceived as noxious is transmitted from the pain receptor to the cord on small, unmyelinated neurons called _____ fibers.

19. Clinical manifestations associated with chronic pain are more _____ than physiologic.

20. Nociception incorporates four interdependent processes, which are

    1. _____

    2. _____

    3. _____

    4. _____

UNIT XII: Case Studies

José is a 21-year-old man who was involved in a motorcycle accident and suffered a closed head injury and spinal cord trauma at the C4 to C5 area. His neck was stabilized in a collar at the scene and he was flown to the emergency department, where he underwent a computed tomography (CT) scan. He is unconscious and is not responding to verbal commands.

1. On admission, a Glasgow Coma Scale assessment is completed. José makes no verbal response, responds to pain by extension (decerebrate posturing), and does not open his eyes to pain. His Glasgow Coma Scale score would be recorded as
   A. 2.
   B. 3.
   C. 4.
   D. 5.

2. This Glasgow Coma Scale rating indicates
   A. a mild head injury.
   B. a moderate head injury.
   C. a severe head injury.
   D. brain death.

3. José's CT scan shows a large hematoma in the subdural space. The most likely source of this bleeding is the
   A. middle meningeal artery.
   B. bridging veins.
   C. circle of Willis.
   D. vertebral artery.

4. José is immediately taken to surgery for evacuation of the hematoma and placement of an intracranial pressure (ICP) monitoring device. José's ICP is to be maintained below 25 mm Hg, if possible. All of the following measures would be expected to reduce ICP *except*
   A. putting the head of the bed down flat.
   B. measures to increase comfort and decrease pain.
   C. mild hyperventilation.
   D. diuretic administration.

5. After his operation, José is prophylactically started on antiseizure medications. The main reason for seizure prevention in this case is the fact that seizures
   A. might compromise the airway and impair respiration.
   B. might cause the intravenous line or ICP monitor to become dislodged.
   C. increase the metabolic activity of the brain and may exacerbate ischemia.
   D. increase the risk of rebleeding of the cerebral hematoma.

6. In the days following his accident, José improves markedly. He returns to consciousness and is able to follow motor commands. However, he is unable to move his extremities. He also has bowel and bladder atony, flaccid paralysis, and a loss of spinal cord reflex activity. These findings are consistent with
   A. autonomic dysreflexia.
   B. spinal shock.
   C. incomplete spinal cord injury.
   D. a good potential for recovery of function.

7. After a few weeks, José's spinal cord reflexes return. José is now at risk for developing autonomic dysreflexia. Signs or symptoms that this problem is occurring would include
   A. tachycardia.
   B. hypotension.
   C. loss of consciousness.
   D. headache and visual changes.

Mrs. Smith is an 84-year-old resident of a long-term-care facility. She has a history of heart failure and is in chronic atrial fibrillation. Her medications include daily Coumadin. She is normally alert and able to accomplish most of her activities of daily living on her own.

8. This morning, Mrs. Smith is still in bed when the aide comes in to check on her. Mrs. Smith is leaning to the right side and drooling from the corner of her mouth. She is unable to respond verbally, and the right side of her body is paralyzed. These signs are most likely a consequence of a
   A. right cerebral stroke.
   B. left cerebral stroke.
   C. lacunar stroke.
   D. global hypoxic stroke.

9. The most important consideration during the acute phase of stroke is
   A. maintaining respiratory and cardiac stability.
   B. determining the location of the stroke.
   C. managing the underlying cause of the stroke.
   D. range-of-motion exercises to prevent complications.

10. Mrs. Smith is taken to the emergency department, where a CT scan is obtained. The purpose of CT scanning at this time is to determine whether the stroke is
    A. hemorrhagic or ischemic.
    B. in the right or left hemisphere.
    C. large or small.
    D. associated with increased ICP.

11. The CT scan shows that there is no significant intracranial bleeding. Considering Mrs. Smith's history and the CT findings, the cause of her stroke is most likely to be
    A. an embolism.
    B. hypertension.
    C. thrombosis.
    D. hypoxemia.

12. Because of the location of Mrs. Smith's stroke, she is likely to experience
    A. left-sided neglect.
    B. impaired vision in the left visual field.
    C. aphasia.
    D. altered sensory function in the left side of the face.

Joe is an 88-year-old man with a long history of Parkinson disease. In the last year, his family has noticed that his ability to care for himself has deteriorated. He rarely engages in activity and often fails to make it to the bathroom in time. His speech has become progressively more difficult to understand.

13. Joe has been taking L-dopa for many years to manage the symptoms of his Parkinson disease. The drug had worked well for a long time, although the dosage had been increased periodically. Joe's family wants to know why he is getting worse instead of better while he is taking his medication. Which of the following statements is the best basis for a reply?
    A. L-Dopa helps prevent the progression of Parkinson disease but can only partially do so.
    B. L-Dopa manages the symptoms only and does not prevent the continued degeneration that occurs with this disease.
    C. There are much better medications for preventing the progression of Parkinson disease than L-dopa, and Joe should be switched to a different medication.
    D. The decline in Joe's status is probably due to a different process because the L-dopa should continue to work indefinitely.

14. Parkinson disease is associated with
    A. a deficiency of dopamine in the cerebral cortex.
    B. an overabundance of dopamine in the striatum.
    C. a deficiency of dopamine in the basal ganglia.
    D. a deficiency of acetylcholine in the brain.

15. Sometimes drugs in combination are more effective than L-dopa alone. Which of the following medications would be appropriate to add to Joe's medications to try to improve his motor function?
    A. An anticholinergic agent
    B. A dopamine-receptor antagonist
    C. An antipsychotic (haloperidol)
    D. Anticholinesterase

16. Which of the following assessment findings would indicate a positive response to the new drug therapy?
   A. An increase in resistance to passive muscle stretch
   B. An increase in movement of the hands while at rest
   C. A faster, propulsive gait while walking
   D. More frequent swallowing and less drooling

17. Joe's family members ask about the likelihood of inheriting Parkinson disease from their father. Which statement about the cause of this disease is the best basis for reply?
   A. Parkinson disease is a familial disorder, and family members should be evaluated.
   B. The cause of idiopathic Parkinson disease is unknown, and no familial pattern has been identified.
   C. Parkinson disease is due to environmental factors only.
   D. Parkinson disease is caused by a virus, and everyone is at approximately equal risk whether they have an affected family member or not.

48 Neurobiology of Psychotic Illnesses

FILL IN THE BLANKS

Fill in the blanks with the appropriate word or words.

1. Altered activity of _____ receptors are associated with the neuropathologic process of schizophrenia.

2. A person who markedly alters his activities of daily living due to the belief that he is being observed by aliens is experiencing _____, whereas a person who proclaims spiders are covering the walls is experiencing _____.

3. Depression that lasts 2 or more years but presents with only one or two symptoms is commonly referred to as _____.

4. The subtypes of bipolar disorder are differentiated in that _____ _____ includes at least one episode of hypomania, but no full manic episode, and a major depression episode, whereas _____ _____ includes at least one episode of full mania.

5. As with schizophrenia, acute psychosis can occur with _____ _____.

6. Part of the neurobiologic basis of schizophrenia is a deficit of the neurotransmitter _____ activity at *N*-methyl-D-aspartate (NMDA) receptors.

7. When individuals are unable to experience pleasure in previously enjoyable experiences, they are said to be experiencing _____.

8. When symptoms of depression develop with exposure to diminished hours of daylight in winter and then abate when daylight hours increase in the spring, the disorder is known as _____ _____ _____.

MULTIPLE CHOICE

Select the one best answer to each of the following questions.

9. Psychotic disorders are characterized by
   A. generalized anxiety.
   B. generalized depression.
   C. altered perceptions of reality.
   D. a personality disorder.

10. Schizophrenia is usually diagnosed during
    A. childhood.
    B. adolescence.
    C. young adulthood.
    D. older adulthood.

173

11. Although the cause of schizophrenia is still unknown, all of the following are thought to be associated with its development *except*
    A. viral infection during the second trimester of gestation.
    B. genetic predisposition.
    C. gestational trauma or malnutrition.
    D. emotional trauma during adolescence.

12. The "negative" symptoms of schizophrenia are difficult to manage and include
    A. hallucinations.
    B. disorganized thinking.
    C. delusions.
    D. flat affect.

13. The "positive" symptoms of schizophrenia are attributed to
    A. excessive activity of dopamine (D_2) receptors in the brain.
    B. excessive activity of norepinephrine receptors in the brain.
    C. insufficient activity of serotonin receptors in the brain.
    D. excessive activity of dopamine (D_1) receptors in the brain.

14. Affective disorders are abnormalities of
    A. personality.
    B. emotion.
    C. reality testing.
    D. social behavior.

15. Major depression is thought to be associated with abnormal brain regulation of
    A. amines, including serotonin.
    B. acetylcholine activity.
    C. glycine activity.
    D. monoamine oxidase activity.

16. Mania is thought to be associated with a relative excess of brain
    A. norepinephrine.
    B. glycine.
    C. acetylcholine.
    D. serotonin.

17. Drugs that may be used to manage depression include all of the following *except*
    A. dopamine receptor antagonists.
    B. serotonin reuptake inhibitors.
    C. tricyclics.
    D. norepinephrine reuptake inhibitors.

18. A patient who experiences periods of reduced sleep and increased activity alternating with periods of low energy and depression is most likely to have
    A. major depression.
    B. bipolar disorder.
    C. schizophrenia.
    D. delusional disorder.

19. Poor impulse control, increased libido, increased appetite, and grandiosity are characteristics of
    A. borderline personality disorder.
    B. anxiety disorder.
    C. mania.
    D. schizophrenia.

20. Mania is commonly managed with lithium, a medication that can impair function of all of the following *except*
    A. cardiac.
    B. liver.
    C. kidney.
    D. thyroid.

21. Tardive dyskinesia is a serious complication of antipsychotic medications and is characterized by
    A. hyperthermia.
    B. coma.
    C. involuntary movements.
    D. depression.

22. Symptoms of psychosis may be associated with all of the following *except*
    A. amphetamine abuse.
    B. anxiety disorders.
    C. dementia.
    D. Alzheimer disease.

23. Delusional disorders are characterized by false beliefs that are
    A. unsystematic.
    B. bizarre.
    C. disorganized.
    D. improbable.

24. Positron emission tomography (PET) scans of individuals with schizophrenia reveal diminished glucose metabolism in what area of the brain?
    A. Frontal cortex
    B. Somatosensory cortex
    C. Temporal lobe
    D. Parietal lobe

25. Examples of positive symptoms of schizophrenia include
    A. flat affect.
    B. hearing voices.
    C. social isolation.
    D. repetitive behavior.

49 Neurobiology of Nonpsychotic Illnesses

FILL IN THE BLANKS

Fill in the blanks with the appropriate word or words.

1. Although anxiety disorders present with similar manifestations, they differ significantly in terms of the _____, _____, and _____ of symptoms.

2. Before an anxiety disorder can be diagnosed, other potential etiologic factors, such as _____ _____ or _____, must be eliminated as the cause of symptoms.

3. Panic disorder is characterized by two types of anxiety behaviors: _____ anxiety and _____ anxiety.

4. The significant and pervasive symptom of generalized anxiety disorder is chronic _____ that leads to a variety of anxiety symptoms.

5. Comorbid conditions often found to be associated with obsessive-compulsive disorder are _____, _____, and _____ _____.

6. Agoraphobia is a rare but debilitating type of _____ _____.

7. In _____ stress disorder hyper-vigilance and intrusive vivid memories are common.

8. Panic disorder incorporates the characteristic manifestations of all anxiety disorders but is distinctive in terms of _____ _____.

9. General anxiety disorder has a _____ onset, and symptoms last for _____.

10. Common types of drugs used to treat anxiety disorders are _____, _____, and _____.

MULTIPLE CHOICE

Select the one best answer to each of the following questions.

11. Nonpsychotic disorders include all of the following *except*
    A. schizophrenia.
    B. phobia.
    C. borderline personality disorder.
    D. post-traumatic stress disorder.

12. Anxiety disorders are characterized by
    A. irrational fears.
    B. poor judgment.
    C. hallucinations.
    D. psychoses.

13. Anxiety disorders include all of the following *except*
    A. panic disorder.
    B. delusional disorder.
    C. obsessive-compulsive disorder.
    D. generalized anxiety disorder.

14. A patient who suddenly experiences overwhelming anxiety accompanied by rapid respiration and heartbeat and a sense of impending doom is likely experiencing a
    A. generalized anxiety episode.
    B. panic attack.
    C. severe obsessive episode.
    D. psychotic break.

15. A person with obsessive-compulsive disorder may feel extremely anxious when
    A. in unclean environments.
    B. performing the compulsive act.
    C. prevented from performing the compulsive act.
    D. distracted from the obsessive thought.

16. Individuals with panic disorder usually have their first occurrence in
    A. childhood.
    B. young adulthood.
    C. middle adulthood.
    D. old age.

17. Manifestations essential to a diagnosis of general anxiety disorder include all of the following *except*
    A. impaired concentration.
    B. uncontrollable worry.
    C. dysphoria.
    D. hypoactivity.

18. Generally, for a diagnosis of attention-deficit hyperactivity disorder (ADHD) to be diagnosed, the onset of symptoms must have occurred prior to age
    A. 2 years.
    B. 5 years.
    C. 12 years.
    D. 20 years.

19. Autism spectrum disorders are defined by a common set of behaviors that includes all of the following *except*
    A. hallucinations.
    B. social communication deficits.
    C. fixated interests.
    D. repetitive movements or behaviors.

20. Which of the following disorders is included in the autism spectrum group of disorders?
    A. Obsessive-compulsive disorder
    B. General anxiety disorder
    C. Asperger disorder
    D. Schizoaffective disorder

Sam is a 29-year-old man with a history of alcohol abuse. He is in the clinic today for complaints of fatigue, weight loss, and insomnia.

1. A review of systems reveals that Sam has a long history of low mood with periods when he feels unable to get up in the morning and misses work frequently. He often does not feel like eating and may go for several days with minimal food intake. He does not think there is much point to his life. In view of this history, which of the following diagnoses is most likely?
   A. Bipolar disorder
   B. Anxiety disorder
   C. Depressive disorder
   D. Personality disorder

2. Sam is interested in learning more about the biochemical alterations that contribute to this disorder. An accurate explanation would be that the pathogenesis is associated with
   A. altered brain serotonin activity.
   B. increased brain norepinephrine levels.
   C. increased activity of D_1 receptors.
   D. increased activity of D_2 receptors.

3. Sam is interested in trying medication to improve his low mood. All of the following medications might be appropriate *except*
   A. selective serotonin reuptake inhibitors.
   B. amitriptyline and other tricyclics.
   C. serotonin and norepinephrine reuptake inhibitors.
   D. benzodiazepines.

4. After taking his medication for 4 days, Sam calls the clinic to report that it does not seem to be helping. Which of the following statements is the best basis for a reply?
   A. Although side effects may occur rapidly, the mood-elevating effect may take 2 or more weeks to occur.
   B. The dosage is probably too low, and Sam should increase the dose.
   C. This medication is unlikely to be effective, and Sam should be switched to another class of medication.
   D. Sam should keep taking the medication, and another medication in a different class should be added.

5. After a month of therapy, Sam is feeling much better. He asks how long he will need to keep taking his medications. Which of the following statements is the best basis for a reply?
   A. Most patients require only temporary therapy, not lasting more than a month or so.
   B. Many patients will require long-term therapy because of the nature of the biochemical alterations in the brain.
   C. These drugs should be discontinued after 1 or 2 months of therapy because of long-term abuse potential.
   D. Once Sam has been able to stop drinking alcohol, he will not need the medication any longer.

Jane is a 44-year-old woman with a history of mood swings that have become progressively more debilitating over the past several years. She is currently in an "up" mood and feels she is doing fine. However, her husband says he is worried because she is spending a lot of money on various things and is not sleeping at night. Sometimes she does not sleep all night and will have just a short nap in the afternoon. She is otherwise physically well and has no other significant past medical history.

6. Jane would most likely be diagnosed with
   A. schizophrenia.
   B. seasonal affective disorder.
   C. bipolar disorder.
   D. dysthymia.

7. A biochemical imbalance thought to contribute to mania is
   A. insufficient brain dopamine.
   B. insufficient brain serotonin.
   C. excessive brain norepinephrine.
   D. insufficient brain acetylcholine.

8. A medication traditionally used to stabilize mood swings is
   A. benzodiazepine.
   B. lithium.
   C. tricyclic antidepressant.
   D. monoamine oxidase inhibitor.

Tom was a 22-year-old pre-law student, studying for the LSAT (law school admission test) to be given in the spring, when he began to exhibit unusual behaviors. He complained of an inability to concentrate, and he was unable to remain in his study group because his divergent thinking was disruptive to other students. He would cock his head as though listening to someone, when no one was speaking. He began to say that he would be given a special version of the examination with only one question because he was such a stellar intellect. He sat cross-legged on the floor of his room for hours, staring into space. His parents were contacted, and they took him to the physician.

9. Based on his history, the most likely explanation for Tom's behavior is
   A. delusional disorder.
   B. personality disorder.
   C. depressive disorder.
   D. schizophrenia.

10. Further assessment of Tom and his family is likely to reveal what risk factor for this condition?
    A. Family history
    B. Preterm labor
    C. History of seizure disorder
    D. Folic acid deficiency

11. If Tom undergoes magnetic resonance imaging (MRI), what findings would be characteristic of his condition?
    A. Increased nicotinic receptors
    B. Diminished sulci
    C. Increased perfusion of the cerebellum
    D. Decreased volume of brain tissue

12. The most likely trigger for Tom's illness is
    A. decreased daylight hours.
    B. group study dynamics.
    C. acute stress from examination anticipation.
    D. childhood abuse.

13. Which of the following medications is likely to help Tom's symptoms?
    A. Antipsychotic medications
    B. Antidepressant medications
    C. Antianxiety medications
    D. Anticholinergic medications

50 Structure and Function of the Musculoskeletal System

MATCHING

1. Match each of the following anatomic terms with the appropriate letter in the figure.

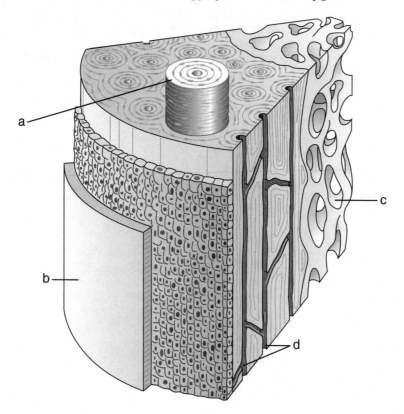

_____ Volkmann canals

_____ Haversian canal system

_____ Periosteum

_____ Cancellous bone

2. *Match each of the following anatomic terms with the appropriate letter in the figure. Some terms may be used more than once.*

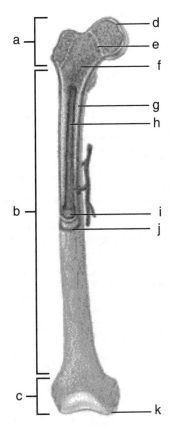

_____ Cancellous/trabecular bone

_____ Epiphysis

_____ Compact/cortical bone

_____ Medullary cavity

_____ Diaphysis

_____ Periosteum

_____ Endosteum

_____ Articular cartilage

_____ Epiphyseal line

Match each of the definitions on the left with its term on the right. Not all terms are defined.

3. _____ Site of linear growth of long bones

4. _____ Cells responsible for deposition of bone

5. _____ Cells responsible for resorption of bone

6. _____ Found at the center of each osteon, where blood vessels and nerves are located

7. _____ Law of bone stresses, which determines deposition and resorption

8. _____ Stage of fracture healing in which callus is replaced by cancellous/ trabecular bone

9. _____ Movable joints

10. _____ Located between the tibia and femur, these structures increase weight-bearing capacity

11. _____ Connective tissues that connect muscles to bone

12. _____ Connective tissues that connect bone to bone

13. _____ Contractile proteins found in striated muscle

14. _____ Ion required for muscle contraction

15. _____ Type of muscle contraction in which no movement occurs

16. _____ A group of skeletal muscles innervated by a single motor neuron

17. _____ Energy storage source for muscle contraction

18. _____ Mature bone cells

19. _____ Protein found in tendons and ligaments

20. _____ Immediate source of energy for muscle contraction

A. Ligaments
B. Consolidation
C. Isometric
D. Adenosine triphosphate (ATP)
E. Actin and myosin
F. Meniscus
G. Epiphyseal plate
H. Trabeculae
I. Ossification
J. Osteocytes
K. Diarthrodial or synovial
L. Calcium
M. Sarcoplasm
N. Motor unit
O. Osteoblasts
P. Creatine phosphate
Q. Wolff's
R. Tendons
S. Haversian canals
T. Elastin
U. Osteoclasts
V. Glucose

FILL IN THE BLANKS

Fill in the blanks with the appropriate word or words.

21. The two primary minerals found in bone are _____ and _____.

22. Hormones influencing bone growth are _____ _____, _____ _____, and _____ _____.

23. As individuals age, muscle cells decrease in both _____ and _____.

24. A train of action potentials in which calcium is _____ into the cytoplasm faster than it is _____ produces a sustained contraction.

25. Receptors for acetylcholine on motor units are of the _____ type.

26. In addition to the production of ATP needed for muscle contraction and relaxation, oxygen is also necessary for the reduction of _____ _____.

27. An increase in temperature results in a/an _____ in conduction velocity across the sarcolemma.

28. Shortening contraction resulting in movement is called a/an _____ contraction, whereas a lengthening contraction is called a/an _____ contraction.

29. At a molecular level, the binding of a myosin head to an actin protein results in the formation of a/an _____.

30. Skeletal muscle is called _____ because of the appearance produced by its arrangement of contractile proteins.

51 Alterations in Musculoskeletal Function: Trauma, Infection, and Disease

TRUE/FALSE

Indicate whether the following statements are true (T) or false (F).

1. _____ All forms of muscular dystrophy have a genetic cause.

2. _____ A comminuted fracture is a result of an injury that produces multiple bone fragments.

3. _____ A partial separation of the articulating surfaces of bones within a joint is called a dislocation.

4. _____ Scoliosis can be detected by observing for uneven alignment of shoulders or hips.

5. _____ The bones are a primary site of tuberculosis infection.

6. _____ Soft tissue injuries heal more rapidly than fractures.

7. _____ Osteomyelitis is most often due to infection by *Staphylococcus aureus*.

8. _____ Damage to supportive soft tissue is the underlying basis of subluxation and dislocation.

9. _____ A compound fracture is one that is smashed, producing multiple fragments of bone.

10. _____ Bone demineralization in multiple myeloma can result in hypercalcemia and pathologic fractures.

FILL IN THE BLANKS

Fill in the blanks with the appropriate word or words.

11. _____ fractures are most commonly seen in childhood, when bone is most flexible.

12. Open fractures are classified based on their _____.

13. Contractile tissue injuries (tendons and muscles) are characterized by _____ _____ _____.

14. Defective bone mineralization due to a deficiency of vitamin D in childhood is called _____, whereas its adult counterpart is called _____.

15. Duchenne muscular dystrophy, the most common and severe form, affects only infants and children of the _____ gender.

16. Myasthenic crisis is an acute exacerbation of myasthenia gravis, whereas cholinergic crisis is usually the result of too much _____.

17. When injured contractile tissues, such as muscles, are moved passively, they may be asymptomatic, but when they are _____ _____, it causes pain.

18. If a joint strain results in a complete tear of the ligament, it is a grade _____ tear.

19. Injury to the anterior or posterior cruciate ligaments results in altered function of the _____.

20. A deficiency of vitamin _____ produces soft bones and is called osteomalacia in adults and rickets in children.

MULTIPLE CHOICE

Select the one best answer to each of the following questions.

21. Ligament injuries are classified by the
    A. degree of tear and joint instability.
    B. amount of pain at rest and with passive range of motion.
    C. amount of weight bearing tolerated.
    D. degree of blood vessel damage.

22. Which of the following statements regarding compartment syndrome is *true*?
    A. A symptom of compartment syndrome is poor muscle tone.
    B. It is due to increased pressure between fascial planes.
    C. It results in impaired fracture healing.
    D. It can be avoided if the fracture is properly aligned.

23. Risk factors for the development of osteoporosis include
    A. male gender.
    B. African American race.
    C. decreased weight-bearing exercise.
    D. previous traumatic fractures.

24. Paget disease differs from osteoporosis in that
    A. only Paget disease has a hereditary component.
    B. osteoporosis is characterized by excessive and abnormal bone growth.
    C. Paget disease can affect the cranial bones.
    D. osteoporosis primarily affects the long bones.

25. The primary reason osteomyelitis is so difficult to manage is that
    A. the origin of the infection is usually elsewhere in the body.
    B. antibiotics that are effective against the causative organisms do not exist.
    C. cysts form around the infection.
    D. it is difficult to attain sufficient antibiotic concentration in bone tissue.

26. The most common malignant tumor of bone is
    A. osteosarcoma.
    B. Ewing sarcoma.
    C. osteochondroma.
    D. chondrosarcoma.

27. The primary symptom of multiple myeloma is bone pain. This is because
    A. nerves in bone are more sensitive than those anywhere else in the body.
    B. excessive plasma cell proliferation erodes the bone structure.
    C. early metastasis to bone is very common.
    D. as the tumor grows, periosteum is destroyed.

28. A major difference between an injury to a ligament and an injury to a tendon is that
    A. ligamental injury typically produces decreased muscle strength.
    B. decreased range of motion is common with tendon injury.
    C. passive stretching of an injured ligament will cause pain.
    D. pain is always greater with tendon injuries because more nerve tissue is involved.

29. All muscular dystrophies have in common
    A. a childhood onset.
    B. a slow onset.
    C. weakness of muscles.
    D. the same specific muscles that are affected.

Chapter **51** **Alterations in Musculoskeletal Function: Trauma, Infection, and Disease**

30. Which of the following statements regarding myasthenia gravis is *true*?
    A. It typically presents with weakness of the large muscle groups of the legs.
    B. It is a neuromuscular disease that has its onset in late middle age.
    C. It is due to excessive production of acetylcholinesterase, resulting in decreased amounts of acetylcholine.
    D. It is a progressive autoimmune disease affecting voluntary muscle function.

31. Fibromyalgia syndrome is characterized by
    A. specific, objective signs on laboratory examination.
    B. emotional instability best managed with psychotherapy and mood-altering drugs.
    C. chronic muscle pain, stiffness, and fatigue.
    D. increased muscle stretch reflexes and muscle spasms.

32. What is the complication called when a fracture has not healed after 6 months?
    A. Delayed union
    B. Malunion
    C. Nonunion
    D. Disunion

33. The presence of callus formation on a bone indicates
    A. osteoarthritis.
    B. early stage of healing.
    C. bone infection.
    D. osteoporosis.

34. Tumors originating in bone
    A. are less common than metastases from other sites.
    B. most frequently affect the elderly.
    C. typically are malignant rather than benign.
    D. originate in the Haversian canals.

35. Osteoporosis is typically defined as a bone density score of
    A. 1.0 standard deviations above the mean.
    B. 2.5 standard deviations above the mean.
    C. 1.0 standard deviations below the mean.
    D. 2.5 standard deviations below the mean.

52 Alterations in Musculoskeletal Function: Rheumatic Disorders

TRUE/FALSE

Indicate whether the following statements are true (T) or false (F).

1. _____ Infectious arthritis typically involves multiple joints simultaneously.

2. _____ Ankylosing spondylitis causes vertebral fusion.

3. _____ Pannus is a vascular scar tissue formed in rheumatoid arthritis that can erode joint tissues and cause contractures.

4. _____ Lyme disease is caused by a spirochete whose vector is most often the deer tick.

5. _____ Scleroderma manifestations are all due to increased density of the epidermal layer.

6. _____ Arthritis results in more disabilities than any other musculoskeletal disease in the United States.

7. _____ Both polymyositis and dermatomyositis are due to bacterial infections of muscle tissue.

8. _____ Infection of a prosthetic joint generally requires its removal.

9. _____ The bleeding into joints seen in patients with hemophilia stimulates inflammation of the synovial tissue.

10. _____ The pattern of joint involvement with psoriatic arthritis is variable from person to person.

FILL IN THE BLANKS

Fill in the blanks with the appropriate word or words.

11. CREST is a syndrome associated with scleroderma, where the letters stand for _____, _____ _____, _____ _____, _____, and _____.

12. Acute rheumatic fever is an inflammatory disease that may develop following a throat infection in which the causative organism is _____ _____ _____ _____.

13. The cause of fibromyalgia syndrome is _____.

14. _____ rash is often found in the multisystem disease known as systemic lupus erythematosus (SLE).

15. The causative organism of infectious arthritis is most frequently _____ _____.

16. Ankylosing spondylitis primarily affects the vertebrae and the _____ _____.

17. The initial systemic manifestations of Lyme disease are similar to the _____.

18. The arthritic manifestations associated with patients diagnosed with the inflammatory bowel diseases _____ _____ and _____ _____ are referred to as enteropathic arthritis.

19. *Compare and contrast rheumatoid arthritis with osteoarthritis by filling in the table with "yes" or "no" to indicate the presence of the specific characteristic on the left.*

Characteristic	Rheumatoid Arthritis	Osteoarthritis
Systemic manifestations		
Inflammatory disease		
Symmetric presentation		
Pain at rest		
Laboratory abnormalities		

MULTIPLE CHOICE

Select the one best answer to each of the following questions.

20. Osteoarthritis
    A. is an inflammatory disease of the joints.
    B. presents bilaterally in a symmetric distribution.
    C. is characterized by remissions and exacerbations of symptoms.
    D. causes the development of osteophyte spurs.

21. Untreated septic/infectious arthritis may result in
    A. ankylosis of the joint.
    B. amputation.
    C. prosthetic joint replacement.
    D. septicemia.

22. In addition to affecting diarthrodial joints, rheumatoid arthritis can also affect
    A. cardiac tissues.
    B. smooth muscle.
    C. ligaments and tendons.
    D. endocrine glands.

23. A characteristic manifestation of SLE that worsens during exacerbations or with exposure to ultraviolet light is
    A. arthralgia and synovitis.
    B. renal failure.
    C. butterfly facial rash.
    D. pleural effusions.

24. Adults who had acute rheumatic fever as children may come to the hospital because of
    A. residual joint manifestations.
    B. replacement of a mitral valve.
    C. a severe rash resulting in dermal abrasions.
    D. a total hip replacement.

25. Individuals who are susceptible to developing Lyme disease are most likely to be exposed while
    A. rock climbing.
    B. hiking or camping.
    C. water skiing.
    D. downhill skiing.

26. The underlying pathologic process of gout is
    A. infection with a bacteria.
    B. painless joint trauma.
    C. muscle injury resulting in myoglobin release.
    D. impaired metabolism of uric acid.

27. Juvenile rheumatoid arthritis
    A. presents in late adolescence or the early 20s.
    B. is managed with acetaminophen (Tylenol) to reduce inflammation.
    C. differs from rheumatoid arthritis in that there is no systemic involvement.
    D. may cause significant joint damage.

28. Patients with rheumatoid arthritis may complain of symptoms of Sjögren syndrome, such as
    A. dryness of the mouth and eyes.
    B. diarrhea.
    C. hypertension.
    D. skin rashes.

29. In the majority of patients with rheumatoid arthritis, laboratory testing reveals a/an
    A. elevated eosinophil count.
    B. normal white blood cell count.
    C. positive rheumatoid factor.
    D. decreased red blood cell sedimentation rate.

30. Scleroderma
    A. is a multisystem inflammatory disease.
    B. affects only the epidermal layer of the skin.
    C. is more commonly found in men than in women.
    D. initially appears in adolescence.

31. All of the following are true statements regarding ankylosing spondylitis *except*
    A. the tendency to develop it is inherited.
    B. it has an acute onset, which is relieved by rest.
    C. it is immune mediated.
    D. it can result in decreased depth of respirations.

32. The exact cause of enteropathic arthritis is unknown, but it is hypothesized to be
    A. exposure to environmental toxins.
    B. latent viral infection.
    C. increased sensitivity with age.
    D. cross-reaction of the immune system with bacterial antigens.

33. Neuropathic osteoarthropathy
    A. is only associated with upper motor neuron disease.
    B. involves motor, sensory, and autonomic nerves.
    C. may develop secondary to diabetes mellitus.
    D. presents with joint inflammation without damage to bone.

34. Reactive arthritis, or Reiter syndrome,
    A. is limited to joint involvement.
    B. has its onset in childhood.
    C. may follow a sexually transmitted infection in men.
    D. usually affects the phalanges joints.

35. Narrowing of the joint spaces of weight-bearing joints is a characteristic x-ray finding in
    A. osteoarthritis.
    B. rheumatoid arthritis.
    C. gouty arthritis.
    D. psoriatic arthritis.

T.G. is a 58-year-old woman who arrives at the clinic for a routine annual physical examination. She says she has been generally in good health this past year, but recently she has noticed increased stiffness in her joints in the morning when she gets up and some swelling in her knees and wrists. Her nurse practitioner suspects rheumatoid arthritis.

1. To meet the criteria for diagnosis of rheumatoid arthritis, additional questions the nurse practitioner might ask could include
   A. "Have these problems been ongoing for a month?"
   B. "How long does the stiffness last?"
   C. "Have you noticed an increase or decrease in your weight?"
   D. "Have you had any injury to your joints recently?"

2. A diagnostic test result that would be indicative of rheumatoid arthritis would be
   A. a bone density scan revealing increased porosity of bone.
   B. an x-ray showing joint erosion of the wrists.
   C. rheumatoid proteins in the urine.
   D. bacteria in the blood.

3. The joints most commonly affected by rheumatoid arthritis are
   A. intervertebral joints in the thoracic region.
   B. one of the hip joints.
   C. hand and wrist joints.
   D. weight-bearing joints.

4. As rheumatoid arthritis advances, a common finding is
   A. flexion contractures.
   B. pathologic fractures.
   C. pain at rest.
   D. loss of tissue elasticity.

5. T.G. is concerned about whether this condition might affect her children. Which of the following statements is the best basis for a reply?
   A. "There is a genetic predisposition to the disease, but it is most likely if you have any sons."
   B. "There's no evidence that the condition is inheritable."
   C. "Rheumatoid arthritis is not inheritable; the condition is caused by a systemic response to an infection."
   D. "If you have daughters, the family history increases their risk."

Thirty-five-year-old B.N. has had SLE for the past 5 years. Her treatment currently focuses on supportive interventions and monitoring for the progression of her disease.

6. As an autoimmune disease, the underlying pathologic process of SLE is
   A. a genetically based hypersensitivity to environmental stimuli.
   B. increased sensitivity to allergens.
   C. deposition of immune complexes in tissues.
   D. an abnormal immune response to infection.

7. The involvement of other organs and the signs and symptoms associated with their diminished functioning are associated with
   A. tissue ischemia and necrosis due to impaired oxygen-binding capacity.
   B. calcification of tissues.
   C. invasion of organ basement membranes by immune complexes.
   D. fluid deposition in tissue spaces interfering with nutrient transport.

8. The most common musculoskeletal manifestations of SLE are
   A. joint pain, swelling, and tenderness.
   B. dislocations and subluxations.
   C. stress fractures.
   D. tendon ruptures and ligamental tears.

9. Both morbidity and mortality in patients with SLE are usually associated with
   A. chronic kidney disease.
   B. early development of atherosclerotic heart disease.
   C. central nervous system involvement causing strokes.
   D. Raynaud phenomenon.

K.K. is 76 years old and is healthy for his age. He wears glasses to read and should begin considering a hearing aid, but his primary complaint is osteoarthritis. He finds that joint pain is getting in the way of gardening, which is his passion.

10. Osteoarthritis
    A. is less common than rheumatoid arthritis.
    B. is not an immune inflammatory disease.
    C. involves hand and wrist joints predominantly.
    D. is bilateral in presentation.

11. A common finding in the physical examination of a patient with osteoarthritis that is not seen in rheumatoid arthritis is
    A. joint swelling.
    B. morning joint stiffness.
    C. crepitus with movement.
    D. joint contractures.

12. Interventions that could be beneficial in managing K.K.'s pain could include
    A. increased weight-bearing activities.
    B. steroid therapy.
    C. acetaminophen.
    D. isometric exercises.

13. A key pathophysiologic feature of osteoarthritis is
    A. the formation of osteophyte spurs.
    B. autoantibody formation.
    C. production of inflammatory cytokines.
    D. synovial proliferation.

R.E. is 10 years old and came to the urgent care center after falling from his bicycle after his dad tightened the hand brakes. His dad thinks R.E. might have broken his arm. R.E. is otherwise healthy, normal in his growth and development, and has no allergies.

14. Of particular concern when a child breaks a bone is a
    A. greenstick fracture.
    B. displaced fracture.
    C. fracture just below the metaphysis.
    D. fracture near the epiphyseal plate.

15. An x-ray reveals an oblique fracture of the radius. An oblique fracture is caused by
    A. a rotational force.
    B. a break near the attachment of a ligament.
    C. a crushing injury.
    D. demineralization of the bone.

16. R.E.'s fracture is a simple fracture. If it were a compound fracture, a major concern would be
    A. prolonged healing of the fracture.
    B. infection.
    C. abnormal healing producing deformity.
    D. impaired callus formation.

17. R.E.'s fractured arm is immobilized with a full-length cast. With a new cast and possible continued swelling from the injury, R.E. will be monitored for the development of compartment syndrome. Signs or symptoms of compartment syndrome include all of the following *except*
    A. decreased movement of the hand and fingers.
    B. the hand or fingers are cold to touch.
    C. decreased sensation of the hand or fingers.
    D. a capillary refill time of less than 2 seconds.

18. It is important to identify compartment syndrome early because if treatment is not promptly initiated,
    A. nonunion of the fracture is likely.
    B. long-term pain management is necessary.
    C. irreversible tissue necrosis occurs.
    D. risk of infection increases.

Forty-five-year-old W.S. is visiting her physician for an annual check-up. Because her 72-year-old mother has significant osteoporosis, W.S. is asking if there are steps she might take to decrease the likelihood of developing this condition.

19. The underlying pathologic process of osteoporosis is
    A. increased osteoclastic activity in the face of decreased osteoblastic activity.
    B. loss of cortical bone while cancellous bone remains intact.
    C. increased osteoblastic activity in the face of decreased osteoclastic activity.
    D. collapse of the Haversian canals.

20. Risk factors for osteoporosis in women include all of following *except*
    A. small bone structure.
    B. Caucasian or Asian race.
    C. use of nonsteroidal anti-inflammatory drugs.
    D. decreased estrogen following menopause.

21. A patient with significant osteoporosis may have
    A. a decreased serum calcium level.
    B. gingivitis.
    C. decreased height from previous measurements.
    D. decreased muscle stretch reflexes.

22. Prolonged immobility can produce osteoporosis because
    A. there is increased renal excretion of calcium.
    B. blood flow to the bone is diminished.
    C. parathyroid hormone secretion is decreased.
    D. decreased weight-bearing stress impairs osteoblastic activity.

23. Suggestions to W.S. that will decrease the risk for development of osteoporosis include all of the following *except*
    A. decreasing alcohol ingestion.
    B. adequate vitamin D and calcium intake.
    C. weight loss.
    D. walking and weight-bearing activity.

24. Prevention of osteoporosis is especially important to prevent related fractures in all of the following locations *except* the
    A. vertebrae.
    B. wrists.
    C. hips.
    D. cranium.

192

53 Alterations in the Integumentary System

MULTIPLE CHOICE

Select the one best answer to each of the following questions.

1. The epidermis is composed of
   A. hair follicles.
   B. nails.
   C. sebaceous and apocrine glands.
   D. stratified squamous epithelium.

2. The predominant cell type in the epidermis is the
   A. keratinocyte.
   B. basal cell.
   C. histiocyte.
   D. melanocyte.

3. Sebaceous glands are stimulated to produce oil by
   A. the sympathetic nervous system.
   B. androgenic hormones.
   C. exercise and increased body temperature.
   D. increased skin blood flow.

4. Piloerection is stimulated by
   A. the sympathetic nervous system.
   B. androgenic hormones.
   C. exercise and increased body temperature.
   D. the parasympathetic nervous system.

5. The primary regulator of skin blood flow is
   A. the parasympathetic nervous system.
   B. body temperature.
   C. autoregulation.
   D. the baroreceptors.

6. The skin is able to regulate body temperature through increased sweating. Sweating is stimulated by
   A. the sympathetic nervous system.
   B. the parasympathetic nervous system.
   C. autoregulation.
   D. activation of sebaceous glands.

7. In addition to providing a barrier to microbial invasion, the outer surface film of dead skin cells is important for
   A. maintaining body temperature.
   B. preventing excessive drying of the skin.
   C. secreting sweat.
   D. sensory perception.

8. Sebaceous glands are most active during
   A. infancy.
   B. childhood.
   C. adolescence.
   D. adulthood.

9. Young children and elderly persons produce less
   A. sweat.
   B. melanin.
   C. keratin.
   D. nail growth.

10. All of the following changes occur in the skin of elderly persons *except*
    A. thinning of the epidermis.
    B. decreased elasticity of the dermis.
    C. decreased vascularity of the dermis.
    D. increased subcutaneous fat.

11. Which of the following statements regarding hair loss is *false*?
    A. Baldness is inherited from the mother.
    B. Only men develop recession of the hairline at the forehead.
    C. Hair loss with aging also affects other areas of the body.
    D. Maximal hair distribution occurs at the age of 40 years and then begins to decline.

12. Changes in the nails associated with aging are primarily due to
    A. decreased blood flow.
    B. reduced dietary protein.
    C. increased production of keratin.
    D. progressive accumulation of lipofuscin.

13. Dark-skinned individuals rarely develop
    A. alopecia.
    B. basal cell carcinoma.
    C. vitiligo.
    D. seborrheic dermatitis.

14. The underlying pathologic process in the development of pressure ulcers is
    A. lack of sufficient tissue blood flow.
    B. prolonged immobility.
    C. inadequate nutrition.
    D. profound dehydration.

15. Which of the following statements regarding scabies is *false*?
    A. The causative organism is a mite.
    B. Scabies is contagious, requiring close personal contact with an affected person.
    C. Scabies is associated with poor personal hygiene.
    D. The predominant symptom is intense itching.

16. Skin manifestations of drug reactions usually include
    A. a few discrete papules on the extremities.
    B. a widespread pruritic rash.
    C. large halo lesions on the back and trunk.
    D. small asymptomatic macules.

17. In children, the lesions associated with atopic dermatitis are usually found on
    A. flexor areas such as the antecubital space and behind the knee.
    B. the scalp along the hairline.
    C. the hands and between the finger webs.
    D. the palms of the hands and soles of the feet.

194

18. Which of the following neoplastic disorders of the skin carries the worst prognosis?
    A. Basal cell carcinoma
    B. Squamous cell carcinoma
    C. Melanoma
    D. Senile keratoses

19. *Vitiligo* is a term that describes a
    A. patch of skin with excessive fine hair growth.
    B. depigmented patch of skin.
    C. hyperpigmented area of skin.
    D. lichenified area of skin.

20. Pallor is best assessed by examining the nail beds, lips, and
    A. underside of the tongue.
    B. palms of the hands.
    C. earlobes.
    D. conjunctivas.

21. Often associated with repeated insulin injections, lipodystrophies appear as
    A. raised palpable nodules.
    B. areas of hyperpigmentation.
    C. smooth, large depressions.
    D. rough, thickened areas.

22. Excessive hair growth is
    A. associated with excessive estrogen.
    B. common in Native Americans.
    C. called hirsutism.
    D. indicative of increased peripheral circulation.

23. Spoon nails commonly are a manifestation of
    A. iron-deficiency anemia.
    B. chronic hypoxemia.
    C. an episode of high fever.
    D. heart failure.

24. Immunization is *not* available for
    A. rubella.
    B. measles.
    C. chickenpox.
    D. roseola.

25. Children who present with skin rashes accompanied by fever are most likely experiencing
    A. a parasitic skin infestation.
    B. a viral infection.
    C. an allergic skin reaction.
    D. an idiopathic skin reaction.

26. Which of the following statements regarding pemphigus skin disorders is *false*?
    A. They appear to be autoimmune in origin.
    B. Blisters form on the skin.
    C. Keratinocytes separate from the skin's basement membrane.
    D. They are highly contagious.

27. Adverse skin reactions to drug therapy
    A. most often are treated with antihistamines and topical corticosteroids.
    B. are more common among men than women.
    C. appear within hours of administration.
    D. are most commonly associated with certain antihypertensive agents.

28. Development of Rocky Mountain spotted fever
    A. often includes cardiac involvement.
    B. is treated with antibiotics.
    C. occurs only in the Rocky Mountain range.
    D. is first manifested as a skin rash.

29. Herpes infections
    A. are all treated with systemic antifungal drugs.
    B. do not have subsequent sequelae.
    C. can be quite painful.
    D. are limited to topical lesions.

MATCHING

Match each of the dermatologic disorders on the left with its descriptor on the right. Answers may be used once or not at all.

30. _____ Secondary lesion

31. _____ Macule

32. _____ Papule

33. _____ Nodule

34. _____ Wheal

35. _____ Vesicle

36. _____ Pustule

37. _____ Lichenification

A. Epidermal thickening and rough patches
B. Excessive scar tissue formation
C. Original appearance (unmodified by time or trauma)
D. Lesion has changed from the initial appearance
E. Raised palpable bump 0.5 to 2 cm in diameter
F. Palpable circumscribed bump less than 0.5 cm in diameter
G. Blister larger than 0.5 cm in diameter
H. Elevated lesion containing purulent exudate
I. Flat, nonpalpable spot up to 1 cm in diameter
J. Small blister up to 0.5 cm in diameter
K. Elevated pink edematous lesion
L. Thinning of the skin and dermis
M. Collection of serous exudates and debris on the skin

Match each of the skin disorders on the left with its usual cause on the right. Answers may be used once or not at all.

38. _____ Cold sores

39. _____ Shingles

40. _____ Ringworm (tinea)

41. _____ Impetigo

42. _____ Atopic dermatitis (eczema)

A. Herpes varicella virus
B. Human papillomavirus
C. Herpes simplex virus
D. Fungus
E. *Staphylococcus*
F. Allergic reaction
G. Yeast

TRUE/FALSE

Indicate whether the following statements are true (T) or false (F).

43. _____ A primary lesion retains its original appearance (unaffected by time or trauma).

44. _____ The function of skin glands is unchanged by aging.

45. _____ Increased production of melanin with age results in graying of hair.

46. _____ The human papillomavirus can invade deep into body tissues.

47. _____ Shingles manifests along the dermatomes of the infected sensory nerves.

48. _____ Leprosy is an infectious disease caused by a bacterium.

49. _____ Psoriasis can affect individuals of any age.

50. _____ Although acne vulgaris is not curable, available treatments can be quite effective.

51. _____ Allergic contact dermatitis is a delayed acquired hypersensitivity reaction.

52. _____ Allergic responses to drugs are often apparent as skin manifestations.

FILL IN THE BLANKS

Fill in the blanks with the appropriate word or words.

53. _____ _____ is a yeast that causes throat infection in newborns and may cause systemic infection in immunosuppressed patients.

54. _____ _____ presents as dandruff and cannot be cured, but it can be controlled.

55. In primary syphilis, the ulcerous lesion is called a _____.

56. The most common cause of allergic contact dermatitis is a reaction to _____.

57. Excessive scar tissue is called a _____.

58. Rocky Mountain spotted fever and Lyme disease are both caused by organisms carried by _____.

59. Both topical and systemic _____ may be used in the management of sunburn, depending on severity.

60. In dark-skinned individuals, petechiae may only be visible on the _____ _____ or _____.

54 Burn Injuries

MULTIPLE CHOICE

Select the one best answer to each of the following questions.

1. The most common burn injury in children, accounting for 60% of all burns in children younger than 15 years, is
   A. electric shock injury.
   B. external chemical burn injury.
   C. scald injury.
   D. exposure to flame.

2. Second-degree burns involve the
   A. epidermis only.
   B. epidermis and dermis.
   C. epidermis, dermis, and subcutaneous tissue.
   D. epidermis, dermis, subcutaneous tissue, and underlying muscle and bone.

3. Third-degree burns involve the
   A. epidermis only.
   B. epidermis and dermis.
   C. epidermis, dermis, and subcutaneous tissue.
   D. epidermis, dermis, subcutaneous tissue, and underlying muscle and bone.

4. A burn is classified as major if it covers more than
   A. 10% of the body surface of a child.
   B. 15% of the body surface of an adult.
   C. 20% of the body surface of a child or an adult.
   D. 25% of the body surface of an adult.

5. The best way to extinguish flames on a burning individual is by
   A. dousing the flames with water.
   B. rolling the individual on the ground.
   C. smothering the flames with a blanket or cover.
   D. using a standard fire extinguisher.

6. Major burns are commonly associated with burn shock, in which there is
   A. excessive edema and fluid volume overload.
   B. significant hemorrhage and anemia.
   C. massive capillary leakage and volume deficit.
   D. rapidly developing sepsis.

7. Topical rather than systemic antibiotics are the preferred treatment for burn injury because
   A. the infecting organisms are entering through the skin.
   B. the burned area is poorly vascularized.
   C. the required antibiotics are available only in topical form.
   D. intravenous access is difficult to establish.

8. Hypothermia and frostbite are also classified as
   A. first-degree burns.
   B. antiburns.
   C. radiant injuries.
   D. thermal injuries.

198

9. The zone of burn injury composed of minimally injured tissue that usually recovers normal function within 1 week is the
   A. zone of stasis.
   B. zone of hyperemia.
   C. zone of ischemia.
   D. zone of equilibrium.

10. Inhalation injury is identified by all of the following *except*
    A. cough.
    B. singed nasal hair.
    C. copious clear sputum.
    D. respiratory stridor.

11. Which of the following groups has a high risk for burn injury?
    A. Children under 4 years of age
    B. Individuals living in apartment complexes
    C. Individuals of Hispanic descent
    D. Individuals living in the suburbs of large cities

12. First-degree burns
    A. often result in pigmentation changes.
    B. are characterized by pallor in response to pressure.
    C. may result in dehydration in infants and elderly persons.
    D. usually heal within 10 to 14 days.

13. The early period of burn shock occurring during the first 24 hours is associated with
    A. leaky capillaries throughout the body.
    B. hyperdynamic cardiac activity and increased cardiac output.
    C. multisystem organ failure.
    D. a reduction in liver production of albumin.

14. Manifestations of carbon monoxide poisoning include all of the following *except*
    A. ketoacidosis.
    B. headache.
    C. nausea.
    D. seizures.

15. Acute management of contact chemical burns should begin with
    A. chemical neutralization.
    B. removal of contaminated clothing.
    C. submersion in tepid water.
    D. identification of the chemical.

16. The fluid that is initially used for fluid resuscitation following burns is
    A. 5% dextrose in water (D_5W).
    B. albumin.
    C. normal saline.
    D. lactated Ringer solution.

17. The most common source of bacteria causing burn wound infection is
    A. transfer from equipment in the room.
    B. cross-contamination from other patients.
    C. the patient's own body.
    D. food and water.

18. Burn wounds requiring grafting preferably will be treated with
    A. xenografts.
    B. allografts.
    C. homografts.
    D. autografts.

19. For patients with severe burns, the focus of nutritional support is the maintenance of the body's
    A. protein.
    B. fat.
    C. carbohydrates.
    D. water.

20. African Americans and Caucasians with red hair
    A. have minimal scar tissue formation.
    B. tend to form keloids.
    C. develop hyperpigmented scars if exposed to sunlight.
    D. form scar tissue more slowly.

FILL IN THE BLANKS

Fill in the blanks with the appropriate word or words.

21. In most home fires, the cause of death is _____ _____.

22. After healing following major thermal injury, the skin is quite dry because of a decrease in the production of _____.

23. Systemic antibiotics are not used to prevent burn wound infection, because the burned tissue has poor _____ _____.

24. The time of greatest risk for infection following grafting burn wounds is the _____ day after surgery.

25. The common assessment tool _____ _____ is an inaccurate indicator of oxygen saturation in carbon monoxide poisoning.

26. Management of the discomfort experienced during the washing of burn wounds is most effectively accomplished with _____.

27. Because of advances in treatment, more than 50% of children with burns covering more than _____ % of their total body surface area will survive.

28. The most common type of burn in children is _____ injury.

29. Hypermetabolism following burn injury is due to the release of large amounts of _____.

30. After burns heal, sweat glands change their normal function and become _____.

31. Burn wound care includes the removal of necrotic tissue, which is known as _____.

32. Fourth-degree burns are often the result of thermal injury due to _____.

33. Airway edema resulting in airway obstruction is typically not clinically identifiable for _____ to _____ hours following burn injury.

34. Skin grafting is necessary for burns of _____ degree or greater.

35. Using the Rule of Nines, a person with a burn involving the inside of one arm and chest would have a/an _____% burn.

36. Physiologically, carbon monoxide poisoning develops because carbon monoxide preferentially binds to _____.

37. Acute renal failure may occur in burns where damaged muscle releases _____ into the bloodstream, producing _____.

38. Following significant burn injuries, the immune system is _____.

39. Burned skin is called _____.

40. _____ _____ are used to help foster flat healing of burn scars.

UNIT XV: Case Studies

B.N. is a 9-year-old girl brought to the clinic by her mother for evaluation of an itchy skin rash. There is no significant medical history and no known allergy. A review of systems reveals only that B.N. reacts excessively to mosquito and other bug bites, which sometimes cause swelling of the lips and face; however, there has never been any respiratory difficulty associated with these reactions.

1. The skin lesions show evidence of chronic scratching and are thickened and scaly. These lesions would be classified as
   A. primary lesions.
   B. secondary lesions.
   C. macules.
   D. papules.

2. The physical assessment findings indicate probable eczema. In assessing the skin, the nurse is aware that the location especially likely to have lesions in this disorder is
   A. behind the knee.
   B. around the ankles.
   C. on the shoulders.
   D. on the scalp.

3. In addition to topical corticosteroids, an important therapy for eczema is
   A. application of drying gels.
   B. frequent bathing in very warm water.
   C. frequent application of skin moisturizers.
   D. application of occlusive dressings.

4. B.N. asks what is causing the itchy rash. Which of the following statements is the best basis for a reply?
   A. The cause of eczema is unknown.
   B. Eczema is thought to be a kind of allergic reaction.
   C. Eczema is secondary to a nervous habit of frequent scratching.
   D. Eczema is simply a dry skin condition.

5. B.N.'s mother is concerned that the topical corticosteroid might have dangerous side effects. Which of the following statements is the best basis for a reply?
   A. The side effects of topical corticosteroids are similar to those of oral corticosteroids.
   B. When used as prescribed, topical corticosteroids have minimal systemic effects.
   C. The only side effect of topical corticosteroids is thinning of the skin.
   D. Topical corticosteroids can be used only for 1 week to avoid serious side effects.

6. Itching (pruritus) is the most disturbing feature of eczema (atopic dermatitis). Should the usual interventions be unsuccessful, which of the following systemic treatments should be considered?
   A. Antihistamines
   B. Antibiotics
   C. Steroids
   D. Barbiturates

7. Understandably, both B.N. and her mother are concerned that they will have to deal with the eczema for the rest of B.N.'s life. They will be relieved to know that
   A. the prescribed interventions should cure the condition.
   B. the condition will likely go into remission and will not recur for months at a time.
   C. in nearly half of the cases, the condition improves with age.
   D. once the source of the allergy is determined, it can be avoided.

C.Y. is a 6-year-old boy who suffered a scald injury on his arm and chest when he fell into a bathtub that was filling with hot water. His parents quickly submerged the burned area in cold water and then brought him to the emergency department.

8. On arrival at the emergency department, C.Y. is crying and says the burned area is painful. The skin is blistered in several areas and the skin is sloughing in others. The burn is categorized as a second-degree burn. This means that
   A. only the epidermis is damaged.
   B. only the epidermis and dermis are damaged.
   C. the epidermis, dermis, and subcutaneous tissue are damaged.
   D. the sensory receptors in the skin have been destroyed.

9. The burn is estimated to cover about 8% of the total body surface area. This means that the risk for burn shock is
   A. high.
   B. low.

10. The parents are concerned about whether they did the right thing in submerging C.Y. in cold water after the burn. Which of the following statements is the best basis for a reply?
    A. "Yes, cold water is a good way to decrease the pain, although it may not reduce the degree of burn."
    B. "Yes, cold water is the best way to extinguish a burn and reduce the degree of burn."
    C. "No, simply applying a wet cloth to the burn would avoid damage to the burned area."
    D. "No, tepid water would be more effective and less of a shock to the skin."

11. C.Y.'s second-degree superficial burn does not require grafting, because
    A. sufficient dermis is available.
    B. there does not appear to be any infection.
    C. he is otherwise healthy.
    D. the size of the involved area is small.

12. C.Y.'s parents are instructed to apply burn cream to the burn twice daily and to observe for signs and symptoms of infection. They are told to seek medical attention in the event of
    A. failure of the burn to heal within a week.
    B. oozing of serous fluid from the blistered areas.
    C. sloughing of skin from burned areas.
    D. progressive swelling and redness of the skin surrounding the burn.

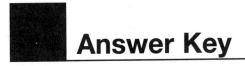

Answer Key

CHAPTER 1

True/False

1. T
2. T
3. F
4. T
5. T
6. T
7. F
8. F
9. F
10. T
11. T
12. F
13. T
14. F
15. T

Multiple Choice

16. D
17. C
18. A
19. A
20. D
21. C
22. A
23. B

Fill in the Blanks

24. populations
25. idiopathic

26. iatrogenic
27. pandemic
28. latent; incubation
29. exacerbation; remission
30. valid
31. circadian rhythm; diurnal variation
32. sensitivity; specificity

CHAPTER 2

True/False

1. T
2. T
3. F
4. T
5. T
6. F
7. T
8. F
9. T
10. T
11. F
12. F
13. T
14. T
15. F

Compare/Contrast

16. (See textbook Figure 2-3 for more examples.)

Physiologic System	Stress-Induced Disease Process
Nervous system	Nervous tic; fatigue; anxiety; depression; insomnia; headaches
Cardiovascular system	Abnormal heart rate, rhythm; hypertension; stroke; coronary heart disease
Gastrointestinal system	Gastritis; irritable bowel syndrome; ulcerative colitis; Crohn disease
Genitourinary system	Irritable bladder; sexual dysfunction; menstrual irregularity
Integumentary system	Hair loss; rashes
Respiratory system	Hyperventilation; asthma; frequent upper respiratory infections
Immune system	Immune deficiency; autoimmune disease; frequent infections
Endocrine system	Hyperglycemia; diabetes mellitus
Musculoskeletal system	Muscle tension headache; backache; autoimmune and inflammatory joint disorders; fibromyalgia

Multiple Choice

17. C
18. C
19. A
20. D
21. B
22. A
23. B
24. C
25. A

Fill in the Blanks

26. nervous; endocrine; immune
27. memory
28. cortisol
29. adaptation; coping
30. Endorphins
31. coping mechanisms
32. glucose
33. cellular; humoral
34. hypothalamus

UNIT I: CASE STUDIES

1. C

Once a stress-related disorder is present, the alarm stage has passed and resistance has not been achieved. Symptom emergence is not a part of Selye's model of stress.

2. D

Once identified, avoiding exposure to a known stressor may prevent triggering of the stress response. Avoiding treatment may contribute to progression of the stress response. It is not helpful to recommend elimination of the stressor or more effective coping, because often these are not possible or not under the individual's control.

3. B

The perception of a stressor and one's physiologic state greatly affect responses. Although migraines can be triggered by stress in susceptible individuals, the degree of stress is not linearly related and neither are all migraines stress related. Although the patient may benefit from better coping skills, the suggestion that her sister's are better than hers as the reason for her migraines is not correct.

4. B

Catecholamines include epinephrine and norepinephrine, which are released during acute stress and acute pain. They bind to β receptors in the heart to increase the heart rate and bind to α receptors to increase the blood pressure. The other hormones do not directly affect the heart rate or blood pressure.

5. A

Excessive cortisol secretion over time may inhibit various aspects of immune competence and predispose to more frequent infectious illnesses. Susceptibility to infections is not known to be related to endorphins or pain medications. Chronic, inadequately treated pain is likely to trigger stress-related problems.

6. B

A primary function of cortisol is to elevate blood glucose levels through hepatic mechanisms. An acute decrease in physical activity might contribute to elevated blood glucose in insulin-dependent diabetes, but this is an unlikely reason in a nondiabetic individual. Pain medications are not known to have direct effects on blood glucose metabolism.

7. D

Distraction from a non–life-threatening stressor can reduce physiologic stress responses; however, the stressor itself is not resolved. This is not the stage of exhaustion, which implies the onset of physiologic dysfunction. Coping strategies that reduce stress responses, and do not produce harm, can be considered effective.

UNIT II

CHAPTER 3

Matching

1. b, i, k, c, e, g, a, j, d, l, h, f

True/False

2. F
3. T
4. T
5. F
6. F
7. T
8. T
9. T
10. F
11. T
12. T

Multiple Choice

13. B
14. C
15. A
16. B
17. B
18. D

Fill in the Blanks

19. proton gradient
20. integrin
21. osmotic
22. three
23. electrochemical
24. gap junctions
25. interstitial; bloodstream

CHAPTER 4

True/False

1. T
2. F
3. T
4. T
5. F

Multiple Choice

6. D
7. B
8. B
9. D
10. B
11. A
12. C
13. B
14. A
15. D

Fill in the Blanks

16. functional reserve; adapt
17. proteins
18. immune response
19. calcium
20. necrosis

CHAPTER 5

True/False

1. F
2. T
3. F
4. T
5. F

Multiple Choice

6. B
7. D
8. D
9. C
10. D
11. C
12. C
13. A
14. B
15. A

Fill in the Blanks

16. 19,000
17. sugar-phosphates
18. transcription
19. stem
20. epithelial, connective, muscle, nerve
21. GTACCATGCCTTAA; GUACCAUGCCUUAA
22. DNA polymerase; RNA polymerase
23. 20
24. epigenetic
25. charged, polar, nonpolar

CHAPTER 6

True/False

1. T
2. F
3. F
4. F
5. T

Multiple Choice

6. A
7. D
8. C
9. D
10. D
11. C
12. D
13. B

Matching

14. D
15. D
16. A
17. A
18. C
19. B
20. D
21. B
22. E

205

Fill in the blanks

23. crossover
24. nondisjunction
25. short; long
26. zero

CHAPTER 7

True/False

1. F
2. T
3. T
4. F
5. F
6. T
7. T
8. F
9. T
10. T
11. F
12. F

Multiple Choice

13. D
14. A
15. C
16. D
17. D
18. C
19. D
20. C
21. D
22. A
23. B
24. B

Compare/Contrast

25.

Characteristic	Benign Tumors	Malignant Tumors
Conventional terminology	Suffix "oma"	Suffix "carcinoma" or "sarcoma"; also leukemia, lymphoma, melanoma
Histology	Similar to tissue of origin; well differentiated	Anaplastic, with abnormal cell sizes and shapes; poorly differentiated
Proliferation rate	Generally slower rate of cycling	Generally rapid rate of cycling
Metastasis	Never; strictly local	High rate of metastasis
Necrosis within the tumor	Rare	Common
Recurrence after treatment	Rare	Common
Prognosis	Good	Poor if untreated or detected at late stage

UNIT II: CASE STUDIES

1. B
Cystic fibrosis is a single-gene defect on chromosome 7 that follows an autosomal-recessive pattern of inheritance.

2. C
There is a one-in-four chance that a given offspring would receive the defective gene from both parents and be affected. There is a two-in-four chance that an offspring would receive only one mutant CF gene and then would be a carrier.

3. A
The risk of bearing an affected child is very low because the child will receive a normal CF gene from the father. The child could be a carrier but is unlikely to be significantly affected because the disease trait is recessive. However, the child could have a spontaneous gene mutation after conception, so the risk is not zero, but it is close to it.

4. A
Down syndrome (trisomy 21) is detected by the presence of three chromosomes 21 in fetal cells and cannot be determined prior to conception.

5. B
Down syndrome is usually associated with the presence of three chromosomes 21; however, this result does not mean that other congenital or genetic defects are not present.

6. A

Prostate-specific antigen (PSA) is a tumor marker for prostate cancer. It is not completely specific for cancer and may be elevated by inflammation of the prostate; however, it is not useful in diagnosing prostate infection. PSA does not differentiate between metastatic and localized cancers; this must be done by further testing, including prostate histologic and staging procedures.

7. A

A biopsy procedure is used to obtain a sample of cells for evaluation but is not inclusive of the entire prostate, surrounding tissue, or possible nodal involvement; therefore, it cannot be used to determine the stage. All of the incorrect answers are data from staging procedures, not histologic procedures.

8. B

Anaplasia means that the examined cells are not well differentiated and demonstrate a variety of cell shapes, sizes, and properties that are not consistent with normal prostate cell morphologic findings. Anaplasia is associated with malignant cell behaviors. Histologic testing cannot determine whether the tumor has spread to distant sites; it can only predict the likelihood that it will do so.

9. C

The N0, M0 designation indicates an absence of node involvement and no evidence of metastasis. The tumor is still localized with a T1 classification, but this does not mean it is benign.

10. D

Radiation is not selective for tumor cells and will affect all cells in the irradiated area; those with more rapid cell division will be more significantly affected. Radiation disrupts DNA and triggers apoptosis, particularly in cells that have less time for repair because they are rapidly dividing.

11. C

Most heritable forms of cancer are associated with the loss of tumor suppression gene activity. The tumor suppression genes normally function to suppress cell proliferation or are part of the DNA repair mechanisms. Oncogenes and proto-oncogenes contribute to cancer occurrence, but they are not usually inherited and they occur as somatic mutations after conception.

12. C

The great majority of breast cancers are not associated with *BRCA* gene abnormalities or other known inherited genetic disorders. The best way to determine if cancer is present is by evaluation of the mass.

13. C

Anaplastic cells are consistent with the presence of a malignant cancer; however, a staging procedure is necessary to determine whether the cancer is localized or metastatic.

14. B

The presence of tumor cells in regional nodes (N2) means that the tumor is not localized (in situ); however, the M0 designation indicates no evidence of metastasis. There is no indication of disease in the other breast.

15. A

Cancer cells are more susceptible to chemotherapeutic agents in certain phases of the cell cycle. Less toxic doses of drugs can be used if they are given over several cycles, thereby reducing damage to normal cells.

UNIT III

CHAPTER 8

Matching

1. E
2. C
3. A
4. G
5. G
6. C
7. A
8. D
9. F
10. C

Multiple Choice

11. B
12. C
13. B
14. D
15. A
16. B
17. A

Fill in the Blanks

18. population
19. reservoir, portal of exit, mode of transmission, portal of entry, host susceptibility

20. fomite
21. disrupted skin or mucous membranes, very young or old, immunosuppression, poor nutrition, chronic illness
22. colonization
23. bacteria, fungi, viruses, parasites
24. viruses
25. physiology

CHAPTER 9

Labeling

1. See textbook Figure 9-2 to check your answers.
2.

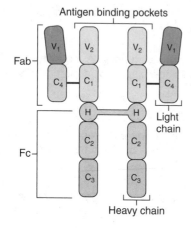

True/False

3. T
4. F
5. T
6. T
7. T
8. T
9. F
10. T
11. T
12. T
13. F
14. T
15. T
16. F
17. T

Multiple Choice

18. C
19. C
20. A
21. C
22. D
23. A

24. B
25. B
26. A
27. B
28. B
29. C
30. B
31. D
32. B
33. A
34. C
35. D
36. B
37. D
38. D
39. B
40. C
41. A
42. B
43. C

Fill in the Blanks

44. Fc (IgG); C3b (complement); toll-like; LPS (CD14) (and others, e.g., mannose receptors)
45. IgE

Matching

46. d, b, a, e, c

CHAPTER 10

Matching

1. C, E
2. A
3. B, E
4. B
5. D
6. C
7. B, E
8. C, E
9. A
10. B, E

Multiple Choice

11. A
12. D
13. A
14. D
15. A
16. B
17. C
18. B
19. A

Fill in the Blanks

20. II, III
21. infection; stress
22. Plasmapheresis; autoantibodies
23. II; antibodies
24. P; S; S; P; P; P

CHAPTER 11

True/False

1. T
2. F
3. T
4. F
5. F

Multiple Choice

6. A
7. A
8. B
9. A
10. C
11. C
12. A
13. D
14. C
15. B

Fill in the Blanks

16. stage (or location)
17. M; M; L; M; M; L; L
18. benzene, cigarette smoke, bioflavonoids
19. anemia, thrombocytopenia, leukopenia
20. autologous; allogeneic

CHAPTER 12

Matching

1. a, e, i, d, h, c, g, b, f

True/False

2. T
3. F
4. T
5. T
6. F

Multiple Choice

7. B
8. C
9. A
10. B
11. C
12. B
13. D
14. B
15. C

Fill in the Blanks

16. 1
17. Nucleoside reverse transcriptase inhibitors, non–nucleoside reverse transcriptase inhibitors, protease inhibitors, integrase inhibitors, co-receptor inhibitors
18. 200
19. reservoirs
20. clinical latency

UNIT III: CASE STUDIES

1. A

Bee-sting allergy usually occurs in response to an IgE-mediated degranulation of mast cells. This occurs when an excessive amount of IgE is produced in response to exposure to bee venom. The IgE binds to mast cells, making them hypersensitive to bee venom. This type of reaction is called anaphylactic, or type I, hypersensitivity.

2. B

Release of inflammatory mediators, particularly histamine, from mast cells produces most of the signs and symptoms of a type I hypersensitivity reaction. IgE does not fix complement, and type I hypersensitivity reactions are not autoimmune. Although eosinophils are often elevated in allergic individuals, they do not produce the typical signs and symptoms of an allergic reaction.

3. D

Epinephrine is effective as an acute treatment for type I hypersensitivity reactions to bee stings because it binds to B_2 receptors in bronchioles and may inhibit bronchoconstriction. It also stimulates the heart to help maintain the blood pressure, which may fall because of vasodilatory effects of histamine. Epinephrine also helps reduce further the release of inflammatory mediators from mast cells. Epinephrine does not bind to or block histamine receptors; antihistamines have this effect.

4. B

Desensitization therapy is effective in reducing the degree of reactivity to bee stings in some individuals. Chronic exposure to small amounts of bee venom is thought to reduce the production of IgE in favor of IgG. All of the other immunosuppressive therapy choices would perhaps suppress the immune response but are associated with excessive adverse effects.

5. C

Plasma cell myeloma (multiple myeloma) commonly invades and degrades bone, causing bones to weaken and be more susceptible to fracture. The degradation of bone is related to an elevated level of serum calcium. An elevated serum calcium level is a common finding in many cancers and is a nonspecific finding, but with the presence of bone involvement, plasma cell myeloma is most likely. Leukemia may cause bone pain because it exerts pressure within the marrow, but it does not usually cause extensive bone degradation. Lymphoma usually presents with enlarged lymph nodes. Osteoporosis is unlikely in a 58-year-old male and is not usually associated with high serum calcium levels.

6. B

Plasma cell myeloma is associated with excessive production of one kind of antibody from the malignant clone of plasma cells. This can be detected by protein electrophoresis, which demonstrates a high concentration (spike) at the position of the monoclonal antibodies. An elevated white blood cell (WBC) count is nonspecific and usually associated with infection or leukemia. A high blast cell count is associated with leukemia. Plasma cells are differentiated cell types and not blast cells. Reed-Sternberg cells are diagnostic of Hodgkin lymphoma.

7. B

Plasma cells are differentiated B cells, which secrete antibody. Although the disease is called myeloma, it is a lymphocytic malignancy (not a myeloid malignancy); therefore, granulocytes and monocytes are incorrect answers.

8. A

The goal of therapy for HIV is to reduce the viral load to undetectable levels. This finding indicates a desired response to therapy; however, it is highly unlikely that the virus has been cleared from the body, so continued therapy is indicated.

9. B

When the CD4 count drops below 200 cells/μL, the Centers for Disease Control and Prevention (CDC) categorizes the disease as acquired immunodeficiency syndrome (AIDS). However, with current treatment options, human immunodeficiency virus (HIV) infection has become a chronic condition with significant longevity for many individuals. Although Ken's immune response is compromised and he is more susceptible to opportunistic infections, it is incorrect to assume that he is unable to mount any immune response.

10. C

The risk of transmitting HIV through sexual contact can be reduced by abstinence, condom use, and therapy to reduce the number of viruses in body fluids. Spermicidal ointments are not effective agents to kill HIV.

11. B

Prep is appropriate only for HIV negative individuals with high risk of exposure, for example through intravenous drug use or sexual transmission.

UNIT IV

CHAPTER 13

Matching

1. H
2. P
3. K
4. L
5. E
6. T
7. I
8. D
9. B
10. G

11. U
12. C
13. F
14. J
15. A

Multiple Choice

16. D
17. A
18. B
19. C
20. C
21. A
22. D

Fill in the Blanks

23.

Anemia Disorder	MCV	MCHC
Iron deficiency	D	D
Aplastic	N	N
Vitamin B_{12} deficiency	E	N
Folate deficiency	E	N
Thalassemia	D	D
Hemolytic	N	N
Acute blood loss	N	N
Erythropoietin deficiency	N	N

24. glycolysis
25. bilirubin
26. 1.34
27. $20; Cao_2 = (Pao_2 \times 0.003) + (Hb\ g/dL \times 1.34 \times Sao_2)$. Sao_2 is entered as a decimal, not %.
28. 25
29. secondary polycythemia; polycythemia vera
30. Bilirubin; conjugated

CHAPTER 14

True/False

1. T
2. T
3. F
4. F
5. T

Multiple Choice

6. C
7. D
8. A
9. A
10. D
11. B
12. B
13. D
14. C
15. D

Fill in the Blanks

16.

Hemostasis Disorder	Platelet Count	PT/INR	aPTT	Bleeding Time
Idiopathic thrombocytopenic purpura	D	N	N	E
Hemophilia A or B	N	N	E	N or E
Liver disease	N or D	E	N or E	E
Aspirin use	N	N	N	E
DIC	D	E	E	E

17. glycoprotein IIb/IIIa
18. cyclo-oxygenase
19. extrinsic; intrinsic
20. ecchymosis; hematuria

CHAPTER 15

True/False

1. T
2. F
3. T
4. T
5. F
6. T
7. F
8. F
9. T
10. T

Multiple Choice

11. D
12. C
13. D
14. D
15. B
16. A
17. C
18. A
19. C
20. B
21. A
22. D

Fill in the Blanks

23. decrease; increase
24. 60
25. increase; decrease
26. 16
27. two
28. increased distending pressure, increased radius, decreased wall thickness
29. 3
30. resistance

CHAPTER 16

True/False

1. F
2. T
3. T
4. F
5. F
6. F
7. T
8. T
9. F
10. F

Multiple Choice

11. D
12. D
13. C
14. A
15. B
16. C
17. D
18. A

Fill in the Blanks

19.

Category	Systolic (mm Hg)	Diastolic (mm Hg)
Normal	<120	<80
Prehypertension	120–139	80–89
Hypertension, stage 1	140–159	90–99
Hypertension, stage 2	≥160	≥100

20. Modifiable: smoking, hypertension, lipid risks, diabetes, obesity, physical inactivity, hypercoagulable (thrombogenic) state. Nonmodifiable: age, gender, family history, ethnicity

21.

Error	Effect on Blood Pressure
Blood pressure cuff too large	Falsely low
Arm positioned above heart	Falsely low
Arm unsupported	Falsely high
Less than 1 minute between readings	Falsely high

22. 90
23. 1, 90
24. heart, kidney, brain
25. heart rate, stroke volume, systemic vascular resistance

UNIT IV: CASE STUDIES

1. D

Iron deficiency anemia is most likely because her red cell indices indicate a microcytic hypochromic anemia. Her age and gender (likely menstruating) fit the profile of iron deficiency anemia. Folate and vitamin B_{12} deficiency produce a macrocytic anemia, and aplastic anemia is usually normocytic and normochromic.

2. B

The large majority of oxygen is carried to tissues in the bloodstream bound to hemoglobin. Each gram of hemoglobin carries 1.34 mL of oxygen per 100 mL of blood when fully saturated, so when hemoglobin falls, the oxygen-carrying capacity of the blood falls accordingly. Anemia does not increase oxygen consumption or affect hemoglobin affinity for oxygen.

3. D

The most likely explanation, given the history and red cell indices, is iron deficiency anemia, which usually results from chronic blood loss. For her age and gender, menstruation is the usual cause. All of the other answers are unlikely because they would produce a normocytic anemia.

4. A

During a period of iron deficiency, the production of new red blood cells (RBCs) is low and the reticulocyte count (immature RBCs) is lower than normal. With reintroduction of iron into the system, the reticulocyte count will improve if iron deficiency was the original problem. An elevated total iron-binding capacity (TIBC) indicates iron deficiency, as does an increased red cell distribution width (RDW). Although the serum iron level will likely increase with iron administration, this does not mean it is being effective in treating the anemia.

5. B

Hemophilia A is caused by a defective gene for clotting factor VIII, which is located on the X chromosome. The disease is recessive, in that a female with one normal factor and one defective factor VIII gene does not express the disease. Males have only one X chromosome and so express the disease when they inherit a defective gene. Hemophilia B is associated with factor IX deficiency and is called Christmas disease.

6. D

Because of his hemophilia, J.K.'s clotting cascade is impaired and he is susceptible to excessive bleeding with minor trauma. Aspirin is an irreversible cyclo-oxygenase inhibitor that permanently inhibits platelet aggregation for the life of the platelet and would further increase the bleeding time. Tylenol does not affect platelets or the clotting cascade. Antibiotics and calcium supplementation would not impair clotting or platelet function.

7. A

In active children who tend to fall and bump themselves, bleeding into joints is a risk. Anemia and purpura may also occur but are not generally due to increased activity.

8. D

A deficiency of factor VIII (hemophilia A) or factor IX (hemophilia B) will prolong the activated partial thromboplastin time (aPTT) because both are operative in the intrinsic pathway of the coagulation cascade, which is measured by the aPTT. The factor VIII level is reduced, not elevated, in hemophilia. The prothrombin time/International Normalized Ratio (PT/INR) test and platelet count should be normal in hemophilia.

9. C

Idiopathic means that the cause of the platelet deficiency is unknown. Many idiopathic disorders are thought to be autoimmune, but the pathophysiology of autoimmunity is still poorly understood. In this case, antibodies are formed against the individual's own platelets, and the antibody-coated platelets are removed and destroyed by the spleen. The liver does not produce platelets. The bone marrow does, and aplastic anemia can be associated with a reduced platelet count, but that is not the problem in idiopathic thrombocytopenia. Aspirin inhibits platelet function but does not usually reduce the number of platelets.

10. A

Unless there is a large amount of bleeding associated with the platelet deficiency, which is unlikely, the hemoglobin usually remains stable. All of the other answers may occur with low platelet numbers and represent bleeding into tissues from prolonged bleeding times associated with minor pressure or trauma.

11. B

A prolonged bleeding time with normal clotting cascade tests (PT and aPTT) is indicative of a platelet disorder. If the PT or aPTT is prolonged, another cause, such as clotting factor deficiencies, must be considered. A decreased red blood cell (RBC) count is a feature of aplastic anemia, but it rarely occurs with thrombocytopenia unless there is hemorrhage.

12. B

According to the National Cholesterol Education Program (NCEP III) criteria, a high-density lipoprotein (HDL) level of more than 40 mg/dL is associated with reduced risk; however, higher is probably better. A goal of 200 mg/dL or less is related to total cholesterol, not HDL.

13. D

Inflammation is a risk factor for development of plaques and for platelet aggregation on plaques. Even those with normal cholesterol levels may benefit from statin therapy.

14. A

Hydrogenated (saturated) fats and trans fats have been associated with heart disease risk in some studies and should be avoided. Animal fats are high in cholesterol and would not be recommended over olive oil. Excessive use of simple sugars and dietary stimulants would pose risks to health.

15. A

It is recommended that individuals with a single high blood pressure reading have it rechecked to avoid a diagnosis based on a spurious reading. Numerous factors, including poor measurement technique, recent exertion, recent cigarette smoking, and anxiety, can cause spurious readings. If the blood pressure is 170/100 mm Hg, treatment is indicated. There is no reason to think that his blood pressure is not really elevated or that the elevation should be attributed to "white coat" phenomenon.

16. D

According to Joint National Committee JNC 7 criteria, a blood pressure reading of 170/100 mm Hg is classified as stage 2 hypertension. Although lifestyle modifications are recommended and beneficial, they are unlikely to be sufficient to control the blood pressure. G.H. has several nonmodifiable risk factors, including age and family history. No information is given to indicate that his hypertension is secondary to any other disorder; however, further evaluation may be needed to rule out this possibility.

17. B

Elevated blood pressure is asymptomatic in most individuals, but it contributes to atherosclerosis, coronary heart disease, stroke, and kidney disease. Treatment will reduce the risk of these complications, but one cannot guarantee that heart attack or stroke will be prevented—one can say only that the risk will be reduced. Untreated hypertension may not progress to higher elevations in blood pressure, nor will treatment cure it. Treatment is for management of blood pressure and risk reduction and will usually need to be continued.

18. C

In addition to elevated blood pressure, retention of fluid leading to edema and leakage of protein into the urine are usually found in pregnancy-induced hypertension (PIH, pre-eclampsia). Nausea, vomiting, fatigue, and lower back pain are common findings in normal pregnancy and are not indicative of PIH. Retinal changes can occur with very high blood pressure, as can rales from heart failure, but her blood pressure is not that high.

19. D

Primary hypertension is most likely. There is no such known diagnosis as postpartum hypertension, and pre-eclampsia occurs only during pregnancy and is not a chronic condition. The thorough workup with no identifiable cause means that secondary hypertension is unlikely.

20. A

Blood pressure is the mathematical product of cardiac output and systemic vascular resistance. In pregnancy, the blood volume and cardiac output increase, which would lead to an increase in blood pressure, except that systemic vascular resistance falls. An increase in heart rate would be expected to increase the cardiac output and, therefore, the blood pressure. Therefore, the only answer that would lead to a decrease in blood pressure is decreased systemic vascular resistance.

UNIT V

CHAPTER 17

Matching

1. a, c, b, d, e, j, i, h, g, f
2. a, g, e, d, c, b, f

True/False

3. T
4. T
5. F
6. F
7. F
8. T
9. T
10. T
11. T
12. F
13. F
14. T
15. T
16. F
17. T

Labeling

18. See textbook Figure 17-7 to check your answers.

Fill in the Blank

19. Phase 0: Influx of Na^+ through fast sodium channels

Phase 1: Cessation of Na^+ influx, beginning of K^+ efflux

Phase 2: Influx of Ca^{2+} through slow calcium channel and continued but slower K^+ efflux

Phase 3: Closure of calcium channels, rapid K^+ efflux

Phase 4: Rest, minimal ionic flux

Multiple Choice

20. A
21. D
22. B
23. A
24. C
25. B
26. C
27. C
28. D
29. B
30. B
31. C
32. C
33. C
34. D
35. C

CHAPTER 18

Compare/Contrast

1.

Characteristic	Myocardial Infarction	Stable Angina Pectoris
Pain character	Severe, crushing, substernal; may radiate to jaw, neck, left arm; patient may have nausea, diaphoresis, sense of impending doom, shortness of breath; may occur at rest or with activity; lasts more than 15 minutes despite rest and/or nitroglycerin	Predictable onset with activity, relieved by rest; usually lasts less than 5 minutes
Electrocardiographic findings	Acute: ST elevation, T wave inversions	May be none; may have transient ST changes during pain
Serum marker elevations	Elevated myoglobin, troponins I and T, CK-MB	No elevations

Multiple Choice

2. D
3. A
4. B
5. B
6. D
7. C
8. A
9. C
10. B
11. A
12. C
13. C
14. A
15. B
16. B
17. D
18. B
19. D
20. B

Fill in the Blanks

21. large lipid core, thin cap
22. stable angina, ischemic cardiomyopathy; unstable angina, myocardial infarction (MI), sudden cardiac arrest; acute coronary syndrome
23. inflammation
24. reperfusion
25. unstable angina
26. NSTEMI (non–ST elevation MI)
27. aspirin
28. Group A β-hemolytic streptococci
29. 50
30. viral
31. cytoskeletal or sarcomere
32. necrotic; electrical
33. age, gender, family history
34. HDL; LDL
35. left circumflex

CHAPTER 19

Multiple Choice

1. D
2. B
3. B
4. A
5. C
6. C
7. D
8. C
9. A
10. D
11. A
12. C
13. C
14. B
15. A

True/False

16. T
17. F
18. T
19. T

20. F

21. T

22. T

23. F

24. F

25. T

Matching

26. C

27. B

28. A

29. E

30. D

CHAPTER 20

Matching

1. C

2. A

3. D

4. B

5. C

6. E

7. C

8. D

Multiple Choice

9. D

10. B

11. B

12. D

13. A

14. B

15. C

Fill in the Blanks

16. progressive

17. cardiac index

18. preload; workload

19. 1500; 2000

20. colloids

21. endotoxin

22. I; IgE

23. decreased; hypoxic or ischemic

24. anaphylactic; septic

25. unresponsive

UNIT V: CASE STUDIES

1. A

Chest pain that occurs predictably with activity and disappears with rest is consistent with stable angina. Although it is happening more frequently, this may be a sign that the plaques are getting bigger or more numerous, but this is still considered stable. Variant angina is usually associated with vascular spasm and occurs unpredictably, often at rest. Unstable angina is associated with clot formation on a plaque and produces symptoms of acute coronary syndrome, which would not predictably disappear with rest. Progressive angina is not a conventional diagnosis.

2. D

Chest pain that occurs at rest and is not relieved within 15 minutes is indicative of acute coronary syndrome, and care should be sought because of the potential to progress to myocardial infarction and dysrhythmia. All of the other answers are attributable to stable angina and do not require immediate evaluation.

3. C

High blood pressure does not reduce coronary perfusion pressure (which is calculated as aortic pressure minus right atrial pressure); increases in aortic blood pressure would therefore actually *increase* coronary perfusion pressure. All of the other answers are true: high blood pressure is a known risk factor for atherosclerosis, increases left ventricular afterload and workload, and contributes to left ventricular hypertrophy (LVH).

4. A

ST elevation on the electrocardiogram (ECG) is an important diagnostic criterion for acute coronary syndrome (ACS); it does not indicate recent myocardial infarction (MI) or impending dysrhythmia, but it also does not rule them out. Other assessments must be made to determine these possibilities.

5. D

Leads II, III, and aVF all view the heart from the inferior angle. ST elevation in these leads is indicative of ischemia in the inferior aspect (apex) of the left ventricle. These leads do not effectively evaluate the septum, anterolateral wall, or right ventricle.

6. A

Acute coronary ischemia is nearly always associated with clot formation in a coronary artery at the site of a ruptured plaque. Therefore, thrombolytic therapy to quickly break down the fibrin of the clot can restore blood flow (reperfusion) and relieve ischemia. Thrombolytics are not known to decrease myocardial oxygen consumption, relax smooth muscle, or reverse the chronic changes of atherosclerosis.

216

7. C

An elevated serum cardiac troponin I level is most specific for myocardial infarction. The total *creatine* kinase measurement and an elevated erythrocyte sedimentation rate (ESR) may accompany myocardial infarction, but they may also occur with numerous other disorders. Creatine phosphate is a form of energy used in cells and is not a marker of cardiac death, although the term is commonly confused with *creatine kinase,* which is the enzyme that produces creatine phosphate, and its cardiac isoform is a marker of cardiac cell death.

8. C

All of the electrocardiograph (ECG) findings listed are normal except for the prolonged PR interval of 0.22 seconds, indicating a first-degree block. A normal PR interval is less than 0.20 seconds. Sinus bradycardia is defined as a heart rate of less than 60 beats/min. There is not enough information to determine if sinus arrhythmia is present.

9. D

A first-degree block is usually well tolerated and does not normally progress to a more serious rhythm; however, continued monitoring is indicated because it is a sign of impaired conduction through the atrioventricular (AV) node. It is not a normal rhythm, but it usually does not require a pacemaker or medications to increase the heart rate.

10. C

Morphine can reduce myocardial oxygen consumption by reducing the preload of the heart. It does this by causing venodilation and pooling of blood in the periphery. If the person is experiencing pain or anxiety, morphine can reduce the sympathetic activation of the heart caused by these symptoms. The other drugs might be expected to improve oxygen delivery to the heart but would not decrease oxygen use by the heart.

11. C

Aortic stenosis and mitral regurgitation are both systolic murmurs; however, with her age and radiation of the murmur to the neck, it is most likely to be aortic stenosis. Mitral stenosis and aortic regurgitation would produce abnormal sounds during diastole, not systole.

12. B

These findings in someone with valvular heart disease suggest left-sided heart failure. This occurs because valve dysfunction creates abnormally high pressures in the cardiac chambers and in the pulmonary capillary bed. Isolated right-sided heart failure would not cause pulmonary congestion; it would present as edema in the systemic circulation. No data suggest pneumonia or acute respiratory distress syndrome (ARDS).

13. B

The ejection fraction is the portion of the end-diastolic volume in the heart (just prior to systole) that is ejected with the heartbeat (stroke volume). It is a measure of the systolic contractile function of the left ventricle.

14. A

An ejection fraction of more than 0.50 in a patient with heart failure is considered to be "preserved systolic function." An ejection fraction of 0.40 is mild systolic dysfunction. Diastolic dysfunction cannot be determined by the ejection fraction, and it is evaluated by dynamics of ventricular filling.

15. B

Several β-blockers have been shown in clinical trials to reduce the death rate in patients with heart failure. Digoxin, nitrates, and diuretics are commonly used in heart failure to manage symptoms but have not been shown to significantly reduce the death rate.

16. C

Hypertrophic cardiomyopathy is the most likely cause of symptoms in a young athlete with no evidence of ischemia on the ECG and a normal blood pressure value. Coronary disease is unlikely at his age and with his activity level. K.K. is not hypertensive, so hypertensive heart disease is unlikely. Myocarditis is an inflammatory condition of the heart that can occur in young individuals and lead to heart failure, but there is no evidence of this in the case information.

17. D

An enlarged septal mass can obstruct the outflow of the aortic valve, particularly during heavy activity, when the cardiac muscle is contracting forcefully. The other conditions listed are not usually associated with septal hypertrophy.

18. C

In a second-degree block, P waves are not reliably conducted through the atrioventricular (AV) node to the ventricle. In a Mobitz type I (Wenckebach) block, the PR interval progressively lengthens until a P wave is not conducted and then starts over again. In this case, the PR interval is consistent, so it would be called a Mobitz type II block. In a first-degree block, the PR interval is prolonged but all P waves are conducted through and associated with a QRS complex. In third-degree block, the P waves and QRS complexes are not related to one another and each occurs at its own pace.

Answer Key

19. B

A second-degree block of this type has a significant risk of progressing to a third-degree block or having a ventricular rate too low to support the cardiac output, so close monitoring and readiness to initiate therapy are indicated. However, if it is asymptomatic, monitoring with no drug treatment is indicated at this time.

20. A

In most cases, hypertrophic cardiomyopathy is associated with abnormalities in sarcomere protein genes and runs in families. Often, the condition is asymptomatic until there is an episode of sudden cardiac arrest, so genetic testing and cardiac echocardiograms of family members are recommended. The outflow obstruction may be improved with surgery, but the cardiomyopathy persists. Progression to heart failure is a risk, as is sudden cardiac arrest, but they are not a certainty. Medications are commonly used to prevent or delay these complications.

UNIT VI

CHAPTER 21

Matching

1. e, a, g, h, c, i, k, d, j, b, f

True/False

2. T
3. F
4. F
5. T
6. T
7. F
8. F
9. F
10. T
11. T
12. T
13. F
14. T
15. T
16. T

Multiple Choice

17. B
18. A
19. D
20. D
21. C

Fill in the Blanks

22. 30
23. hypertension
24. stasis of blood, hypercoagulability, injury to the vessel
25. metastasize
26. smoke cigarettes
27. $P_{AO_2} = 106$; $A - aD_{O_2} = 46$
28. $P_{AO_2} = 235$; $A - aD_{O_2} = 135$; no, the $A - aD_{O_2}$ has increased significantly.
29. vasoconstriction
30. fistula
31. anatomic dead space
32. atelectasis
33. resistance
34. resistance; elasticity
35. medulla, pons

CHAPTER 22

Compare/Contrast

1.

Characteristic	Chronic Bronchitis	Emphysema
Early hypoxemia	Likely	Unlikely
Early CO_2 retention	Likely	Unlikely
Productive cough	Likely	Unlikely
Increased anteroposterior chest diameter	Unlikely	Likely
Cor pulmonale	Likely	Unlikely

Multiple Choice

2. A
3. C
4. D
5. A
6. B
7. C
8. A
9. D
10. A
11. A
12. B
13. C
14. C
15. C
16. A

True/False

17. T
18. F
19. F
20. T
21. T

Fill in the Blanks

22. inflammation
23. resistance
24. decreased; increased
25. chronic bronchitis
26. radial traction
27. emphysema
28. peak flow
29. back blows; Heimlich maneuver
30. bronchial provocation

CHAPTER 23

True/False

1. T
2. T
3. F
4. T
5. F

Multiple Choice

6. D
7. A

8. C
9. B
10. A
11. C
12. A
13. B
14. C
15. B
16. C
17. A

Fill in the Blanks

18. transudates; exudates
19. increased
20. inspiration; expiration
21. Ghon tubercle
22. Bacterial; viral
23. respiratory alkalosis
24. adolescents
25. empyema
26. airborne droplets
27. coronavirus
28. inflammation
29. coal dust
30. functional residual

UNIT VI: CASE STUDIES

1. C
Ventilation and perfusion preferentially distribute to the dependent lung fields. In a patient with pneumonia in the right lung, positioning with the right lung down would send more blood flow to the consolidated, nonventilated areas of the lung and produce a worse V/Q mismatch, which would decrease oxygen diffusion into the blood and produce a lower arterial oxygen saturation.

2. C
The law of 5s is a formula used to estimate what the P_{AO_2} and arterial Pa_{O_2} should be on a given inspired oxygen concentration. This patient is receiving 28%, so taking that times 5 equals 140 mm Hg.

3. A
Hypoxemia is the primary concern. Asthma increases resistance to airflow through the airways and can produce areas in the lungs that do not receive good alveolar ventilation. Pneumonia is associated with consolidation and poor alveolar ventilation. Both conditions lead to a low V/Q ratio and hypoxemia. Asthma leads to increased (not decreased) residual volume. Apnea and weakened respiratory muscles are not consequences of asthma or pneumonia.

4. D
Hyperinflation occurs with obstructive disorders such as emphysema and asthma but not with pneumonia, which is an alveolar consolidation and atelectatic problem. Productive cough and fever are commonly associated with pneumonia. Tachypnea is a response to decreased tidal volume or hypoxemia and can occur with pneumonia.

5. A
Increased temperature (as well as acidemia, hypercarbia, and increased 2,3-bisphosphoglycerate [2,3-BPG]) decreases the affinity of hemoglobin for oxygen. This is termed a *shift to the right* on the oxyhemoglobin dissociation curve.

6. B

The major difference between obstructive and restrictive diseases is that airway resistance and peak expiratory flow rates are maintained in restrictive diseases and are abnormal in obstructive diseases. Compliance is decreased in restrictive disorders and increased in obstructive disorders. Inflammation can occur in both types of lung disease.

7. D

Emphysema typically produces a barrel-shaped chest with an increased anteroposterior dimension. This is thought to be a result of loss of lung parenchyma, resulting in reduced elastic recoil and increased residual lung volume and functional residual capacity. The vital capacity is reduced in emphysema, and the intrapleural pressure is unchanged.

8. C

Dyspnea is the subjective feeling of being unable to "get enough air." This is likely the result of decreased alveolar ventilation and reduced surface area for gas exchange. Patients with emphysema do not usually have much sputum, although those with chronic bronchitis typically do. Nausea and pleuritic pain are not symptoms of emphysema.

9. B

Emphysema results in loss of parenchymal tissue and formation of enlarged alveolar sacs that are weakened by loss of elastin. These blebs are more susceptible to rupture than normal lung parenchyma, which can result in pneumothorax. Cancer, pleural effusion, and tuberculosis are not more common in patients with emphysema.

10. C

Many patients with emphysema are able to maintain a normal arterial oxygen concentration despite a reduced surface area for gas exchange by increasing their minute ventilation. This increased respiratory effort often produces a mild reduction in $PaCO_2$, which is indicative of hyperventilation. This is not necessarily due to an increase in tidal volume, but either an increased tidal volume or increased respiratory rate would increase alveolar ventilation.

11. expiratory; inspiratory

Obstructive disorders such as emphysema are associated with airway collapse on expiration, making the expiratory phase more difficult, whereas patients with restrictive disorders must generate a higher-than-normal inspiratory pressure to overcome their stiff, noncompliant lungs, which resist inflation.

12. D

The $A - aDo_2$ is a measure of the difference between what arterial oxygen should be and what it actually is. The determination of what it should be is based on calculation of what the alveolar oxygen partial pressure should be under given conditions of barometric pressure and inspired oxygen concentration. A widening gap between what arterial oxygen should be and what it actually is indicates a problem with gas exchange in the alveoli and is a good indicator of lung function.

13. A

Cystic fibrosis is a genetic abnormality of the chloride channel that results in abnormal fluid movement into various secretions in the body, including respiratory secretions, pancreatic secretions, and sweat. Decreased fluid content makes these secretions excessively thick, with poor mobility.

14. B

Mucous production in the lung and subsequent sweeping of it out of the respiratory tract by cilia is a protective mechanism against bacterial infection. Cystic fibrosis patients are particularly susceptible to respiratory infection because of loss of this function and accumulation of pockets of mucus, which may allow bacteria to proliferate.

15. D

Chloride ion supplementation would not be helpful. Although the genetic abnormality is with a chloride channel, the problem is not a lack of chloride in the body but an inability to move it into the correct fluid compartments. All of the other choices are commonly employed in the treatment of cystic fibrosis.

16. B

Pneumothorax is a collection of air in the pleural space. A collection of pus is called an empyema; a puncture of the chest wall can produce a pneumothorax but does not necessarily do so.

17. C

The area of lung near a pneumothorax often undergoes atelectasis, either because of a loss of negative pressure in the pleural space or sometimes because of positive pressure in the pleural space that causes compression of the lung. This causes decreased alveolar ventilation in the area, resulting in decreased breath sounds heard over that area of the chest.

220

18. A

The effect of closed chest drainage is to reestablish negative pressure within the pleural space to encourage re-expansion of the affected lung alveoli. These systems also can remove accumulated pleural fluid, but that is not the problem in this patient with a pneumothorax.

19. B

Croup is usually a consequence of upper airway reactions to viral infections. High fever is not usually associated with croup, nor is it a result of immunization.

20. D

Croup is usually a benign problem and does not progress to significant respiratory distress; epiglottitis, however, can result in significant swelling in the area that could obstruct the airway.

21. D

Croup generally affects the upper airway structures, increasing resistance to inspiratory air flow. This causes the child to produce increased negative inspiratory pressures to overcome the obstruction. Because of the pliability of the chest wall in children, retractions of the intercostal muscles may be evident. Expiratory wheezing and a prolonged expiratory phase are typical of increased lower airway resistance, as would occur with asthma. Clubbing is a consequence of chronic hypoxemia and is not seen in an acute disorder such as croup.

UNIT VII

CHAPTER 24

True/False

1. T
2. T
3. T
4. F
5. F
6. T
7. F
8. T
9. T
10. F
11. T
12. F

Completion

13. N
14. N
15. H
16. H
17. L

Compare/Contrast

18.

Characteristic	Hypernatremia	Hyponatremia

Etiologic factor	Chronic diarrhea
	Restricted access to fluid
	Altered thirst sensation
	Diabetes insipidus
	Diabetes mellitus
	Fevers
		Excess hypotonic IV fluid
		Excess ADH (SIADH)
		Excess water intake:
		  Tap water enemas
		  NG irrigation with water
		Psychogenic polydipsia

Clinical findings	High serum sodium
	High serum osmolality
	Confusion, lethargy, convulsions
	  owing to cellular shrinking
		Low serum sodium
		Low serum osmolality
		Confusion, lethargy, nausea, coma, convulsions
		  owing to cellular swelling

Treatment	Increase free water intake Hypotonic IV fluids Treat slowly to avoid rebound cellular swelling	Free water restriction Avoid hypotonic IV fluid Perhaps diuretics Can administer hypertonic IV solutions cautiously

19.

Characteristic	Hyperkalemia	Hypokalemia

Etiologic factor	Increased intake:
	    Accidental IV bolus
	    Salt substitute
	Administration of older units of blood
	Decreased excretion:
	    Oliguric renal failure
	    Low aldosterone
	Shift from body cells:
	    Crushing injuries
	    Acidosis
	    Chemotherapy
		Decreased intake:
		    NPO status
		    Anorexia, vomiting
		Increased excretion:
		    Diuretics
		    High aldosterone
		    Diarrhea, vomiting
		    Nasogastric suction
		Shift into body cells:
		    Alkalosis
		    Glucose/insulin infusion

Clinical findings	Muscle weakness Ascending paralysis Cardiac dysrhythmias	Muscle weakness, cramps Paralytic ileus Cardiac dysrhythmias
Treatment	Dialysis Sodium polystyrene sulfonate (Kayexalate) Insulin/glucose Correct acidosis if present	IV or PO potassium replacement Correct alkalosis if present

20.

Characteristic	Hypercalcemia	Hypocalcemia

Etiologic factor	Increased intake:
	    Excessive antacids
	    Excessive vitamin D
	Decreased excretion:
	    Hyperparathyroidism
	Shift from body cells:
	    Immobility
	    Hyperparathyroidism
	    Malignancy
		Decreased intake:
		    Malabsorption syndrome
		    Milk intolerance
		Increased excretion:
		    Chronic renal insufficiency
		    Hypoparathyroidism
		Shift out of blood:
		    Massive blood transfusion
		    (citrate binding)

Clinical findings	Muscle weakness
	Constipation
	CNS depression
		Muscle cramping, twitching, tetany:
		    + Chvostek sign
		    + Trousseau sign
		Convulsions, laryngospasm

Treatment	Increased fluid intake Manage underlying cause Parathyroidectomy tumor resection Diuretics	IV or PO calcium supplementation

21.

Characteristic	Hypermagnesemia	Hypomagnesemia
Etiologic factor	Excessive antacid intake IV infusion for pregnancy-induced hypertension Renal failure	Malabsorption syndrome Alcoholism Diuretics

Clinical findings	Muscle weakness
	Decreased deep tendon reflexes
	Similar to hypercalcemia
		Muscle cramping, twitching:
		    + Chvostek sign
		    + Trousseau sign
		Similar to hypocalcemia

Treatment	Increased fluid intake Diuretics	IV or PO magnesium replacement

22.

Characteristic	Hyperphosphatemia	Hypophosphatemia
Etiologic factor	Renal failure	Chronic alcoholism Refeeding after starvation High glucose solutions (TPN)
Clinical findings	Precipitation of $CaPO_4$ salts in organs, joints, vessels, etc. Often associated with hypocalcemia	May have multisystem signs and symptoms because of cellular energy failure: phosphate is needed for ATP synthesis
Treatment	Phosphate-binding antacids Diuretics Measures to increase calcium absorption	IV or PO phosphate replacement

Multiple Choice

23. A
24. C
25. C
26. D
27. A
28. C
29. B
30. B
31. D
32. B
33. D
34. B
35. C
36. A
37. B

Fill in the Blanks

38. saline excess (extracellular volume excess)
39. water
40. 3.5; 5.0
41. hypopolarized; a hypopolarized
42. Trousseau; hypocalcemia, hypomagnesemia
43. cancer (malignancy)
44. depression (weakness)
45. reciprocal; decreased; elevated

CHAPTER 25

True/False

1. F
2. T
3. T
4. T
5. F
6. F
7. T
8. T

Completion

9. L
10. N
11. N
12. Abnormality: alkalosis; Origin: respiratory; Compensation: Yes
13. Abnormality: acidosis; Origin: respiratory; Compensation: No
14. Abnormality: acidosis; Origin: metabolic; Compensation: Yes

Multiple Choice

15. D
16. B
17. A
18. C
19. B
20. A

Fill in the Blanks

21. 20:1
22. $NH_3 + H^+ \rightarrow NH_4^+$, $HPO_4^{2-} + H^+ \rightarrow H_2PO_4^-$
23. depression; excitation
24. mixed (combined) acid–base imbalance
25. respiratory alkalosis

UNIT VII: CASE STUDIES

1. A

Low blood pressure while supine, dizziness upon trying to stand, low urine output, and an elevated heart rate are all consistent with a diagnosis of saline (or extracellular fluid) deficit. Hyponatremia must be diagnosed by serum sodium evaluation. Renal failure is a possible consequence of severe prolonged saline deficit, but that is unlikely at this time. The low urine output is because the kidneys are conserving fluid, not because they have failed. Hypovolemic shock is a possible consequence of severe saline deficit, but there is no reason to suspect cardiogenic shock in this case.

223

2. B

A serum sodium of 150 mEq/L is elevated above the normal range (135 to 145 mEq/L) and indicates a water deficit, which is also called hypernatremia. A high serum sodium level does not evaluate saline balance, only water balance.

3. C

Normal saline or another isotonic fluid is most appropriate to increase extracellular and intravascular volume and improve blood pressure and heart rate. This is because saline does not create a change in osmolality of the extracellular compartment, so none of it will move into cells and all of it will stay in the extracellular compartment. All of the other fluid choices are hypotonic and would reduce the osmolality of the extracellular compartment, causing water to move into the cells. This would be less effective in accomplishing the goal of improving the blood pressure and heart rate.

4. C

A drop of 10 mm Hg in blood pressure and an increase of 16 beats/min in heart rate with standing indicate a significant orthostatic change, which is consistent with a saline deficit. Although Joe has received 3 L of isotonic fluid, he needs more isotonic fluid replacement to replenish the saline deficit. He is, however, responding to fluid replacement because his supine heart rate and blood pressure are improved from baseline.

5. D

Vomiting causes loss of gastric secretions, which are rich in H^+, and could lead to a loss of metabolic acids sufficient to cause metabolic alkalosis. Respiratory acidosis and alkalosis are from changes in $PaCO_2$, which would not occur as a direct result of vomiting. Metabolic acidosis would occur with loss of bicarbonate-containing fluids, as with diarrhea.

6. C

Ketones in the blood can produce a metabolic acidosis known as ketoacidosis. This is a fairly common consequence of insulin deficiency, which alters fat metabolism to produce excessive ketones. Ketones can be used as an energy source by many tissues but in excess can produce metabolic acidosis.

7. A

This is a compensated metabolic acidosis. Metabolic acidosis is evident because of the lower-than-normal bicarbonate concentration. Compensation occurs by a reduction in $PaCO_2$. This is a fully compensated metabolic acidosis because the pH is back to within the normal range of 7.35 to 7.45.

8. A

Because the acid–base disorder is compensated, medical measures to change bicarbonate or $PaCO_2$ are likely to do more harm than good and are unnecessary. The $PaCO_2$ is low as a compensatory response and is not the problem, so breathing into a paper bag is contraindicated. The insulin deficiency should be treated, which will stop the production of ketones, and the acid–base problem should then resolve itself.

9. C

Hyperkalemia is a common concurrent problem in ketoacidosis, thought to occur because the liver leaks potassium into the bloodstream under conditions of insulin deficiency. Administration of insulin is usually accompanied by reuptake of potassium back into the liver cells.

10. D

A high blood sugar reading in a type 1 diabetic along with glycosuria indicate that a fluid volume deficit is present. Glycosuria causes osmotic diuresis by the kidney, resulting in large fluid losses. The glucose remaining in the circulation becomes more concentrated with more fluid loss.

11. A

George has a respiratory acidosis, as indicated by the low pH and the elevated $PaCO_2$. The HCO_3^- is higher than the normal range, indicating an effort by the kidneys to compensate. However, the pH needs to get back into the normal range of about 7.35 to 7.40 before it would be called compensated respiratory acidosis.

12. B

Respiratory acidosis is a result of inadequate alveolar ventilation. Although oxygen administration might improve the low oxygen level, it will not help the alveolar ventilation problem. Administration of bicarbonate in this situation is inappropriate because it will contribute to the development of $PaCO_2$, which George is unable to excrete efficiently. Reducing his oxygen supplementation is likely to worsen his hypoxia and will not do anything to improve alveolar ventilation.

13. C

The pH is back within the normal range; however, the HCO_3^- and $PaCO_2$ are still abnormally high, so this is not a normal blood gas measurement. The pH being on the acid side of 7.40 is what helps make the diagnosis of respiratory acidosis rather than metabolic alkalosis. The pH is within the normal range, so it is compensated.

14. A

Increased alveolar ventilation is the key to reducing arterial levels of CO_2. Although an increase in HCO_3^- would improve the pH and the degree of compensation, in this patient the HCO_3^- has remained steady at 30 mEq/L between the first and second blood gas samples, so increased HCO_3^- was not the reason for improvement. Dead spaces are areas that are ventilated but not perfused with blood. This patient had the opposite problem, areas of low ventilation.

UNIT VIII

CHAPTER 26

Matching

1. e, c, i, j, b, g, f, d, a, h, k
2. H
3. I
4. O
5. X
6. E
7. S
8. U
9. L
10. P
11. W
12. C
13. Q
14. G
15. A
16. N
17. F
18. J
19. R
20. D

True/False

21. T
22. F
23. F
24. T
25. T

Fill in the Blanks

26. 5
27. WBC; RBC; tubular epithelial
28. ultrasonography
29. creatinine (or inulin) clearance rate
30. fenestra; slit pores

CHAPTER 27

True/False

1. F
2. T
3. T
4. T
5. F
6. T
7. F
8. T
9. T
10. T

Multiple Choice

11. B
12. D
13. C
14. A
15. B
16. C
17. A
18. D
19. B
20. D
21. B
22. C
23. B
24. D
25. A

Fill in the Blanks

26. struvite
27. glomerulonephritis
28. antibodies
29. protein
30. ultrasonography

CHAPTER 28

True/False

1. T
2. T
3. F
4. F
5. T
6. T
7. T
8. F

225

Multiple Choice

9. C
10. B
11. B
12. A
13. D
14. C
15. C
16. A
17. D
18. D
19. B
20. A

Fill in the Blanks

21. diabetes mellitus
22. ischemia
23. 90
24. erythropoietin
25. nitrogenous

CHAPTER 29

True/False

1. F
2. T
3. F
4. T
5. T
6. T
7. F
8. T
9. F
10. T

Multiple Choice

11. C
12. B
13. B
14. A
15. D
16. D
17. C
18. C
19. B
20. A
21. A

Fill in the Blanks

22. parasympathetic nervous system
23. ureterocele
24. interstitial cystitis
25. urge
26. hematuria
27. peripheral nervous system
28. functional
29. sensitivity
30. structural or congenital

UNIT VIII: CASE STUDIES

1. D

Cystitis is commonly associated with symptoms of dysuria, frequency, and urgency. Bladder tumors are usually asymptomatic, as are bladder calculi. T.G. may also have pyelonephritis, but further assessment, including a finding of costovertebral angle (CVA) tenderness and urinalysis for white blood cell (WBC) casts, would be necessary to make this diagnosis. Other symptoms of pyelonephritis include fever, back pain, and nausea; these are not stated in the case, making it an unlikely diagnosis at this point.

2. A

A urinalysis would be most helpful in diagnosing cystitis. The presence of leukocytes, red blood cells (RBCs), and protein is common, as is the presence of nitrites, depending on the type of infecting organism. The other tests are for structural abnormalities and would be normal and not helpful in the diagnosis of cystitis.

3. C

Most cases of cystitis are associated with bacterial infection. The finding of bacteria in the urine is diagnostic of bladder infection. The other choices relate to findings on the other tests presented in the question, which would not be done to evaluate cystitis.

4. A

Bladder infections are common in sexually active women. Unless they are occurring frequently, in which case a structural problem might be a contributing factor, they are usually treated empirically with a standard course of antibiotics.

5. B

Abstinence from sexual intercourse is not necessary with cystitis. Cystitis is usually caused by *Escherichia coli* from the rectal area and is not a sexually transmitted disease. Measures to avoid contaminating the urethra with colonic bacteria, increased fluids, and frequent urination to flush bacteria from the urethra may be helpful.

6. A

Severe gastrointestinal flu typically causes vomiting and diarrhea, which predispose to a loss of extracellular volume (ECV). Low ECV is a risk factor for prerenal renal failure because perfusion to the kidney can be impaired. Postrenal renal failure occurs with obstructions in the collecting system and would not occur as a result of vomiting and diarrhea. Pyelonephritis and glomerulonephritis can cause intrarenal renal failure but would not be a consequence of the gastrointestinal disturbance.

7. C

The stage of prerenal oliguria occurs when the kidney responds appropriately to signals indicating low blood volume. These include low filtration pressure in the glomerulus and hormones such as angiotensin II, aldosterone, and antidiuretic hormone (ADH) (which increase reabsorption of sodium and water by the renal tubules). Increased sodium reabsorption results in a lower-than-normal urine sodium level, and increased water reabsorption contributes to a high urine osmolality. The blood urea nitrogen (BUN) rises more quickly than the creatinine in conditions of low blood volume, resulting in a ratio of more than 20:1. The finding of low specific gravity would not occur in prerenal oliguria, because that would imply that the kidney is excreting excess water; therefore, this is the correct answer.

8. B

Prerenal oliguria is treated by measures to increase blood flow to the kidneys. Extracellular volume expansion with an isotonic fluid is standard treatment. At this stage, renal failure has not yet occurred and dialysis is not necessary. Monitoring the blood urea nitrogen (BUN) and limiting protein intake would not be helpful treatments. Aggressive diuretic therapy is contraindicated because it would further deplete the extracellular volume and worsen the prerenal renal failure risk.

9. A

As the kidney enters acute renal failure, kidney tubule cells die and slough to form tubular cell casts, which may be found in the urine. This is called acute tubular necrosis (ATN). Hematuria is not a characteristic of ATN. Oliguria means low urine output, so one would not expect to find an increase in urine output during this stage. The concentration of sodium in the urine will usually increase because the tubule cells become dysfunctional and are no longer able to respond to endocrine hormones that were causing sodium retention.

10. A

The glomerular filtration rate (GFR) is most closely associated with the creatinine clearance rate, which determines the serum creatinine level. This is because creatinine is produced at a fairly constant level in the body, is freely filtered by the glomerulus, and is minimally processed by the renal tubule cells. Therefore, the amount cleared by the kidney reflects the amount filtered by the kidney and can be used to estimate the GFR. As the GFR changes, the serum creatinine increases or decreases in a direct relationship.

11. C

Pyelonephritis is usually caused by infective organisms that gain access to the kidney by traveling from the lower urinary tract up the ureters and into the collecting ducts of the kidney. Recurrent or inadequately treated urinary tract infections are the usual cause of chronic pyelonephritis. There may be a structural anomaly, such as malimplantation of the ureters or benign prostatic hyperplasia (BPH), which contributes by causing urinary stasis, but infection of the kidney is the primary cause.

12. D

Chronic pyelonephritis leads to progressive nephron loss over time and is an important cause of chronic kidney disease and renal failure. It is not premalignant and generally does not cause fluid and electrolyte problems, unless is has already progressed to renal failure. Cystitis may precede or be concurrent with pyelonephritis, but pyelonephritis is not likely to cause cystitis.

13. D

Antibiotic therapy is important for treating chronic pyelonephritis. If it is not appropriately prescribed and taken as directed, it could lead to inadequate eradication of bacteria or predispose to bacterial resistance to the antibiotics. The other choices may be issues in homelessness, but they are not as important for treatment of pyelonephritis.

14. Compare/Contrast

Characteristic	Cystitis	Pyelonephritis
Frequency, urgency, and dysuria	Yes	Yes
Increased serum WBCs	No	Yes
Flank pain	No	Yes
Fever	No	Yes
Costovertebral angle tenderness	No	Yes
Urinary casts	No	Yes

15. A

The visceral and colic pain associated with passing calculi through the ureters is commonly associated with nausea and vomiting. Loss of urinary control (enuresis) or decreased urinary output is unlikely. Diarrhea is not a related manifestation.

16. B

If renal calculi are suspected, a plain x-ray of the kidneys, ureters, and bladder area is commonly performed. Most, but not all, stones are radiopaque and will show up on x-ray. Urine culture is generally not helpful, because renal calculi are not usually associated with infection. Serum creatinine and blood urea nitrogen (BUN) levels would not change in the acute timeframe of passing a urinary calculus, and calculi do not often reduce the glomerular filtration rate (GFR). A computed tomography (CT) scan essentially is a more expensive set of x-rays and would generally not be used initially for this reason, although it would be effective in identifying calculi.

17. D

Increased fluids will help move the stones along through increased flow of urine through the ureters. Use of opioid analgesics is often required to control pain and reduce colicky ureteral spasms. Hospitalization and intravenous fluids usually are not required, unless there is associated urosepsis or severe nausea preventing any fluid intake. This would be an unlikely scenario in the case presented. NPO status would be contraindicated, because it would reduce urinary flow. Bed rest would not be necessary, and many individuals with renal colic are unable to stay still in bed because of pain.

18. B

Acute glomerulonephritis has a significant risk of progressing to renal failure because of damage to the glomeruli and renal parenchyma. This type of renal failure would be called intrarenal renal failure. Prerenal refers to a problem with blood flow to the kidney, which does not usually accompany glomerulonephritis. Postrenal refers to a problem in the collecting system, which is not the primary problem in glomerulonephritis. Acute tubular necrosis (ATN) may be a consequence of various types of acute renal failure, but it is not considered one of the primary types.

19. D

A high level of protein in the urine is the initiating factor in nephrotic syndrome. Usually, this occurs at a 24-hour urine protein loss of greater than 3 to 4 gm. At this rate of loss, the liver is unable to synthesize albumin at a rate to replace protein losses, and hypoproteinemia occurs. This contributes to another feature of nephrotic syndrome, generalized edema. Nephrotic syndrome does not occur during the stage of renal failure or acute tubular necrosis (ATN), but it may precede it in some cases.

20. C

Hematuria is not a component of the nephrotic syndrome, although it may occur during the acute phase of glomerulonephritis. Nephrotic syndrome is associated with edema, ascites, and pleural effusion because of the abnormally low colloid oncotic pressure in the blood associated with hypoproteinemia.

21. C

Glomerular inflammation is a common feature of glomerulonephritis, leading to leakiness of the capillary glomerular membrane. This allows protein and red blood cells, which would normally not cross into the urine filtrate, to do so.

22. D

Weak peripheral pulses are not a feature of extracellular fluid volume overload. They might occur with volume deficit or peripheral arterial disease. All of the other choices are symptoms of extracellular volume overload, often associated with heart failure.

23. C

Hypocalcemia is a common feature of renal failure because the kidneys fail to produce activated vitamin D, which then interferes with the absorption of calcium from the diet. In addition, the kidneys are unable to efficiently rid the body of phosphate because of a low glomerular filtration rate, which contributes to hormonal dysregulation associated with hypocalcemia.

24. A

Osteodystrophy is a degenerative condition of the bone that occurs with chronic renal failure as a consequence of low vitamin D levels and overactivity of parathyroid hormone. It takes months to develop and is not usually seen in the short timeframe of acute renal failure. Metabolic acidosis, hyperkalemia, and azotemia are features of both acute and chronic renal failure.

25. B

Chronic kidney disease is a progressive disorder, even when the initiating event may have been resolved. Significant nephron loss tends to progress to further nephron loss through mechanisms that remain largely unknown. The rate of progression is often predictable, following a more-or-less linear course that can be plotted by the rate of increase in serum creatinine levels.

26. D

Individuals with end-stage renal failure have a low glomerular filtration rate (GFR), which makes it difficult to rid the body of fluids, potassium, and nitrogenous waste products; therefore, these substances may be restricted. Nitrogenous wastes are produced by metabolism of proteins. Caloric needs are not reduced as a result of renal failure.

UNIT IX

CHAPTER 30

Matching

1. a, f, g, d, e, c, b

True/False

2. T
3. F
4. F
5. F
6. T
7. F
8. F
9. T
10. T

Multiple Choice

11. B
12. C
13. A
14. C
15. D
16. A
17. B
18. C

CHAPTER 31

Multiple Choice

1. B
2. A
3. D
4. B

5. C
6. D
7. C
8. A
9. B
10. D

True/False

11. T
12. T
13. F
14. F
15. T

Fill in the Blanks

16. seventh
17. infection
18. *Escherichia coli*
19. β-blockers
20. testosterone
21. Peyronie disease
22. diabetes
23. phosphodiesterase type 5
24. infertility
25. eighty

CHAPTER 32

Matching

1. b, e, h, d, c, a, g, f
2. C
3. J

229

4. E
5. M
6. K
7. F
8. L
9. G
10. H

True/False

11. F
12. T
13. T
14. T
15. F
16. T
17. F

Fill in the Blanks

18. endometrium
19. osteoporosis
20. first

CHAPTER 33

Matching

1. B
2. C
3. A
4. E
5. D

Multiple Choice

6. B
7. B
8. D
9. D

10. C
11. A
12. C
13. B
14. D
15. B

Fill in the Blanks

16. cystocele; childbirth
17. protein
18. surgical
19. Papanicolaou (Pap)
20. upper outer

CHAPTER 34

Multiple Choice

1. A
2. A
3. C
4. D
5. B
6. D
7. C
8. B

Fill in the Blanks

9. eyes
10. salpingitis
11. II
12. 3 to 6 weeks
13. genital warts
14. *Chlamydia*
15. immunosuppressed

UNIT IX: CASE STUDIES

1. A
The placenta is the source of hormones that support growth of the fetus and prepare the body for delivery; however, the purpose of hormonal changes of pregnancy are to support the fetus and, in some cases, may be detrimental to the health of the mother, contributing to various discomforts and adverse events during pregnancy.
2. A
Most of the weight gain during pregnancy occurs in the second and third trimesters as the uterus enlarges, fluid volume increases, and fat is deposited. The fetus constitutes a minor portion of the weight gained in most pregnancies; in normal pregnancies, most of the fluid weight is not in the form of edema.
3. D
Significant facial and periorbital edema is not a normal finding of pregnancy and may indicate a generalized edema associated with pregnancy-induced hypertension (pre-eclampsia). The other changes could be expected during a normal pregnancy.

4. C

Iron is poorly absorbed and in increased demand during pregnancy to support increased red blood cell production. Iron is not stored in significant amounts and is difficult to obtain sufficiently in dietary sources, so it is usually supplemented during pregnancy.

5. B

Hot flushes are a common symptom during the perimenopausal phase, when hormone levels are in flux. These flushes often present as sudden warmth and redness of the face and neck.

6. C

At menopause, estrogen production begins to decline as ovarian function declines. Most of the symptoms of menopause can be ameliorated by estrogen replacement therapy, indicating that estrogen deficiency is the source of most symptoms.

7. B

Estrogen enhances bone deposition and inhibits bone resorption. Estrogen deficiency is associated with accelerated bone resorption and is a risk factor for osteoporosis. Although autoimmune disorders and type 2 diabetes are more common with aging, they are not a consequence of declines in estrogen production.

8. C

In women, gonorrhea may have few or no noticeable symptoms. Untreated infections may progress to pelvic inflammatory disease and negatively affect reproductive function. Because both gonorrhea and chlamydial infection are transmitted sexually, they often coexist, but not always. In certain age groups and risk groups, gonorrhea is common.

9. D

Inflammation of the epididymis is a potential outcome of gonorrheal infection in men, and the infection is more likely to be symptomatic in men than in women. Urinary tract infection and Bartholin gland inflammation occur in women.

10. A

Gonorrhea may cause inflammation and pain in the pharynx, causing patients to complain of sore throat.

11. B

Malignant tumors of the breast are often small, nontender nodules that may be fixed in the tissue. Benign fibrocystic lumps are usually less discrete, tender to palpation, and mobile and may wax and wane in size under the influence of menstrual hormone fluxes.

12. B

A family history of breast cancer in the patient's mother or siblings and excess exposure to estrogen because of early menarche, late menopause, and few pregnancies are considered risk factors for breast cancer. There is controversy about the relationship of dietary fat and breast cancer, but a diet of 20% calories from fat is a low-fat diet and would not be considered a risk. Fibrocystic breast lumps are not precancerous and are not thought to increase the risk for breast cancer.

13. D

More than two thirds of breast cancers are found in the upper outer quadrant of the breast. There is usually more breast tissue located in this area.

14. D

The best answer of these choices is the degree of lymph node involvement, which is another way of indicating the stage of the disease. More lymph node involvement is an indicator of malignant potential and the propensity for metastasis.

15. B

An elevated prostate-specific antigen (PSA) level is used as a marker for prostate cancer; however, it is not very specific for the disease and can be elevated in conditions of prostate inflammation. When PSA is significantly elevated, further evaluation for prostate cancer is necessary.

16. C

Stasis of urine can occur with obstruction of the urinary outlet by an enlarged prostate. Chronic urinary stasis from incomplete emptying of the bladder is a risk factor for urinary tract infection. In the absence of obstruction, usually caused by benign prostatic hypertrophy (BPH), urinary tract infection is relatively uncommon in men.

17. C

Benign prostatic hyperplasia is an extremely common finding in men as they age, indicating that to a certain extent it may be a normal finding of the aging male reproductive system.

CHAPTER 35

Matching

1. i, d, h, a, c, b, e, n, j, o, f, m, k, g, l
2. c, a, g, j, i, d, b, e, f, h
3. B
4. B
5. A
6. C
7. B
8. C
9. C
10. C
11. B
12. B

True/False

13. T
14. F
15. T
16. T
17. F
18. T
19. F
20. F
21. T
22. T
23. T
24. F
25. F
26. F
27. F
28. T
29. F
30. T

CHAPTER 36

Compare/Contrast

1.

Characteristic	Ulcerative Colitis	Crohn Disease
Abscess formation	Yes	Yes
Bloody diarrhea	Yes	Yes
Fistula formation	No	Yes
Rectal bleeding	Yes	No
Mucosal layer involvement	Yes	Yes
Transmural involvement	No	Yes

Fill in the Blanks

2. low fiber
3. nonsteroidal antiinflammatory drugs (NSAIDs), alcohol, tobacco
4. Gastric; duodenal
5. volvulus; intussusception
6. megacolon

Multiple Choice

7. D
8. D
9. C
10. A
11. D
12. A
13. D
14. B
15. B
16. C
17. A
18. C
19. D
20. B
21. D
22. D
23. C
24. A
25. C
26. D

CHAPTER 37

Multiple Choice

1. C
2. B
3. C
4. C
5. C
6. A
7. D
8. C

True/False

9. T
10. F
11. T
12. F
13. T
14. T

Fill in the Blanks

15. cystic; hepatic; common bile
16. stasis or hypomotility
17. insulin, glucagon, somatostatin (or amylin)
18. cholesterol
19. lithotripsy, chemodissolution
20. autodigestion

CHAPTER 38

True/False

1. T
2. T
3. F
4. T
5. F
6. F
7. T
8. T
9. F
10. F

Multiple Choice

11. D
12. D
13. B
14. D
15. A
16. C
17. D
18. A
19. A
20. A
21. B
22. C
23. C
24. A
25. B

Fill in the Blanks

26. K; clotting factors
27. albumin; oncotic
28. jaundice
29. bleeding; blood pressure
30. asterixis

UNIT X: CASE STUDIES

1. D
Unconjugated bilirubin is lipid soluble and has a tendency to accumulate in the tissues. Although an increase in unconjugated bilirubin can occur with hemolysis, in this case the most likely cause is impaired liver function associated with cirrhosis.

2. A
The cirrhotic liver becomes sclerosed and fibrotic with reduced channels for blood to flow through it. This creates an obstruction to blood flow from the portal system, which increases capillary pressure behind the obstruction. The portal system drains blood from the entire gastrointestinal tract; therefore, obstruction in the liver can produce increased pressure in the esophageal vessels and elsewhere in the gastrointestinal tract.

3. C
Acute upper gastrointestinal bleeding frequently presents as hematemesis (vomiting of blood). The hematocrit does not drop much until fluids have been replaced, because plasma and red blood cells are lost together. Confusion and coma are common in individuals with hepatocellular failure because these patients do not metabolize certain substances well, but this is not as suggestive of acute bleeding as is hematemesis. Likewise, abdominal distention or abdominal bleeding can be a feature of cirrhosis, but neither is as characteristic of upper gastrointestinal bleeding as is hematemesis.

4. C
Nitroglycerin and octreotide acetate dilate the portal vessels and can reduce portal hypertension. The other choices may be appropriate treatments for esophageal varices; however, they do not decrease portal hypertension.

5. B
One important function of the liver is to synthesize several of the clotting factors that circulate in the bloodstream and participate in the clotting cascade. All of the other choices are also related to abnormal liver function but are not directly related to the problem of excessive bleeding.

6. C
IgM is the first type of antibody to be made by plasma cells upon exposure to a new antigen. Along with the elevated liver enzyme aspartate aminotransferase (AST), its presence indicates an acute infection with hepatitis A virus. If anti-hepatitis A IgG were present, that would indicate past infection, and immunity. Exposure, but no infection, would not produce an antibody response.

7. C

Hepatitis is commonly associated with fatigue, low-grade fever, anorexia, nausea, and generalized discomfort in the area of the liver, which is located in the right upper quadrant, not the left. Acute abdominal pain and pain in the left upper quadrant are not characteristic of hepatitis.

8. D

Hepatitis A is acquired by oral ingestion of contaminated food or water and may be spread from person to person through poor handwashing and handling of food or water that is then ingested by others. This is sometimes called the "oral-fecal" mode of transmission. Hepatitis A is not transmitted by sexual intercourse. Because there is no chronic carrier state for hepatitis A, transmission by contaminated needles or blood is unlikely.

9. D

Of the choices given, abdominal ultrasound would be most helpful in confirming the diagnosis of cholecystitis because it would show whether stones were present in the gallbladder and whether the gallbladder appeared inflamed. The other tests might also be abnormal as a consequence of cholecystitis but are not as helpful in diagnosing the disorder.

10. C

In nearly all cases, cholecystitis is associated with gallstones.

11. B

Cholecystectomy is curative of cholecystitis because the gallbladder is removed and recurrence is therefore impossible. With procedures to break up the gallstones or dissolve them chemically, there is a significant risk of recurrence.

12. A

All of the choices are possible consequences of cholecystitis, but rupture of the gallbladder is the main complication of untreated inflammation of the gallbladder. The combination of an inflamed gallbladder sac and increased internal pressure secondary to gallstones that may be obstructing outflow contributes to the risk of rupture.

13. B

The cystic duct at the outlet of the gallbladder is the most common site of biliary obstruction by gallstones.

14. C

Aspirin and NSAIDs are medications that inhibit the enzyme cyclo-oxygenase, which is important in the production of prostaglandins. These medications are known to impair normal function of the mucosal barrier that protects the epithelial cells in the stomach from the acidic environment of the gastric contents. Most peptic ulcers are associated either with chronic NSAID use or with *Helicobacter pylori* infection.

15. D

Substances that impair blood flow to the gastric mucosa (smoking) or cause chronic mucosal irritation might contribute to gastritis and peptic ulcer disease. Estrogen is not known to have these effects.

16. B

Blocking acid secretion from entering the lumen of the stomach or neutralizing the secreted acid with ingested antacids is a standard therapy for peptic ulcers. These measures will reduce the proteolytic activity of pepsin in the stomach, which is inactivated at a less acidic pH, as well as reduce the damage from the acid itself.

17. B

Pepsinogen is converted to pepsin in the presence of a low pH, which is accomplished in the stomach by secretion of protons by parietal cells in the gastric mucosa. Pepsin is permanently denatured when the pH rises above about 4.0.

18. A

Ulcerative colitis affects only the mucosal layer of the colon, whereas Crohn disease can affect all layers of the bowel and is therefore susceptible to producing fistulas between loops of bowel. Crohn disease can affect the large or small bowel and, because it affects the small intestine, is susceptible to causing malabsorption, whereas ulcerative colitis does not.

19. A

Both Crohn disease and ulcerative colitis are characterized by chronic inflammation of the bowel. The exact cause of these disorders is unclear but may be a form of autoimmunity. Drugs that reduce inflammation or suppress the immune system are mainstays of therapy for both disorders.

20. A

Both Crohn disease and ulcerative colitis usually present in young adulthood. Some of the other choices occur only in Crohn disease (adhesions), and although remissions and exacerbations are common, neither of these inflammatory bowel diseases has a significant chance of full spontaneous recovery. Pus in the stool implies infectious colitis, which is not a characteristic of either disease.

CHAPTER 39

Matching

1. D
2. I
3. E
4. B
5. G
6. A
7. L
8. O
9. K
10. P

True/False

11. F
12. T
13. T
14. F
15. T
16. F
17. T
18. T
19. T
20. F

Multiple Choice

21. A
22. D
23. B
24. B
25. B

CHAPTER 40

Fill in the Blanks

1. acromegaly; pituitary gigantism
2. free water
3. calcium
4. tissue resistance (or receptor dysfunction)
5. elevated (or increased)
6. exophthalmos
7. surgery
8. autoimmune
9. cortisol
10. thyroid storm

Multiple Choice

11. D
12. A
13. C
14. C
15. B
16. A
17. D
18. B
19. A
20. C
21. D
22. B
23. B
24. A
25. D

CHAPTER 41

True/False

1. F
2. F
3. T
4. T
5. F
6. T
7. F
8. T
9. T
10. F

Multiple Choice

11. B
12. D
13. B
14. D
15. A
16. D
17. A
18. C
19. B
20. C
21. C
22. D
23. D
24. B
25. D

CHAPTER 42

Fill in the Blanks

1. anabolism, catabolism
2. age, body composition or size
3. catabolism

4. 7

5. fats, proteins, carbohydrates

6. positive

7. ghrelin, leptin

8. fatty acids

15. A

16. B

17. A

18. D

19. D

Multiple Choice

9. A

10. B

11. A

12. C

13. B

14. C

True/False

20. T

21. F

22. T

23. T

24. T

25. T

UNIT XI: CASE STUDIES

1. B

When the tubular load of glucose exceeds the reabsorptive capacity of the glucose transporters in the proximal tubules, glucose remains in the filtrate; in later segments of the kidney tubule, it acts as an osmotic force to oppose the reabsorption of water. Glycosuria therefore causes polyuria by its osmotic effects. Polydipsia is a response to the loss of excessive fluids in the urine, not a cause of it.

2. C

Excess production of ketones causes a metabolic acidosis called ketoacidosis, resulting in an excess concentration of protons (H^+) in the blood, which is measured as a decreased pH. The compensatory response by the lungs is to reduce the blood $PaCO_2$, not increase it. The other two choices are unrelated.

3. A

Ketoacidosis is a form of metabolic acidosis for which the compensatory response is hyperventilation (to blow off more CO_2), which will increase the pH back toward normal. Hyperventilation does not affect oxygenation of the blood.

4. B

An insulin dosing schedule that most closely mimics the natural response of the pancreas to dietary intake will improve growth and development and reduce complications. Multiple small doses are preferred over fewer larger doses. Alterations in blood flow to different tissues may affect the rate of absorption of insulin injected into different subcutaneous depots. Insulin is more rapidly absorbed from the abdomen than from the arm, leg, or buttock. Insulin sites should be rotated, and in children who dislike having a shot in a particular place, it should be avoided as much as possible. A hot bath or shower after an insulin injection will also increase the rate of absorption and should be avoided. Some children have different responses when insulin is injected into different sites, and this should be monitored; however, most will not notice much difference between alternate sites, and rotation of sites is encouraged.

5. D

The glycosylated hemoglobin, or HbA_{1C}, is a measure of the percentage of hemoglobin that has glucose molecules attached and is an indicator of the red blood cell (RBC) exposure to glucose over the course of the life of the RBC. Typical RBCs circulate for about 3 months, so the HbA_{1C} is a reflection of the average blood sugar over that time. All of the other choices are indicators of acute blood sugar control and can change quickly, within minutes or hours, so are not good indicators of chronic blood sugar control.

6. C

Diagnosis of hypothyroidism in an adult is not from a congenital condition such as cretinism or thyroid dysgenesis, which would have been apparent shortly after birth. Graves disease is a form of hyperthyroidism, not hypothyroidism. Of the choices given, Hashimoto thyroiditis is the most likely cause of adult-onset hypothyroidism.

7. A

Primary hypothyroidism would be evident as a low T_4 level and a high thyroid-stimulating hormone (TSH) level. This is because when the thyroid gland fails to produce thyroid hormone in adequate amounts (primary disorder), the pituitary gland does not receive enough negative feedback from the circulating hormone and releases more TSH in an attempt to stimulate the gland into more production. In contrast, hypothyroidism from pituitary failure (secondary disorder) would be evident as a low T_4 level and a low TSH level. Thyroid-releasing hormone is not typically measured to diagnose hypothyroidism.

236

8. D
Menstrual irregularity is a common occurrence in women with hypothyroidism. Diarrhea and exophthalmos commonly are seen as features of Graves disease, which is associated with hyperthyroidism, not hypothyroidism. Jaundice is unrelated.

9. B
Although the mechanisms that cause type 2 diabetes are still poorly understood, and genetics and aging play a role, the clearest association is with obesity, with about 90% of diabetic patients being overweight. Autoimmune disease is associated with type 1 diabetes but is not thought to be a risk factor for type 2 diabetes.

10. C
In the early phases of type 2 diabetes, most patients are thought to develop a tissue resistance to the actions of insulin. More insulin is produced by the pancreas to overcome this resistance and bring blood glucose levels toward normal. One potential cause of tissue resistance is a defect in the insulin receptors.

11. C
The typical complications of long-standing diabetes are macrovascular (atherosclerotic disease of the coronary arteries, peripheral arteries, and carotid arteries), which predispose to myocardial infarction, peripheral arterial disease, and thrombotic stroke, and an increased risk of kidney disease, neuropathy, and retinopathy. The other choices are not significantly increased with type 2 diabetes.

12. A
Hypertension occurs commonly in patients with type 2 diabetes and may be associated with hyperinsulinemia. Hypertension with or without concomitant type 2 diabetes increases the risk for kidney disease (nephropathy).

13. D
Below-the-knee amputation is a consequence of poor peripheral circulation secondary to peripheral arterial disease. Amputation occurs more commonly in patients with diabetes, in part because of the reduced sensation in the feet secondary to neuropathy. Injuries and infections may go unnoticed by the patient until amputation may be the only option. The other options are common as a consequence of aging, but they are not more common in patients with diabetes.

14. B
Of the choices given, acute adrenocortical insufficiency is the most likely explanation for hypotension, hypoglycemia, and hyperkalemia. Addisonian crisis is an acute condition caused by cortisol insufficiency when the adrenal gland fails. Addison disease is thought to have an autoimmune cause. Thyroid storm and pheochromocytoma would likely cause high blood pressure, not low blood pressure. Diabetic ketoacidosis could explain the low blood pressure and high serum potassium, but the blood sugar would be elevated, not low.

15. D
Correct diagnosis of the problem as glucocorticoid insufficiency in the previous question would lead one to choose administration of glucocorticoid. Addison disease is a life-threatening condition, but it responds well if treated early with glucocorticoid replacement therapy. The other choices are treatments for the other (incorrect) choices in the previous question.

16. B
One important role of the adrenal cortex is to respond to physical and emotional stressors by releasing glucocorticoids. Glucocorticoids help maintain blood sugar and blood volume and work permissively with other hormones, such as catecholamines, to support blood pressure. In Addison disease, the adrenal cortex is unable to secrete cortisol in response to stress, which predisposes to adverse events. When known stressors are anticipated, such as an elective surgery or during infectious illness, the administered dose of glucocorticoid is usually increased.

17. C
Chronic systemic glucocorticoids are associated with a number of adverse effects, including osteoporosis, fragility of capillaries, disorders of collagen synthesis in the subcutaneous tissue, suppressed immune responses, and loss of muscle tissue.

18. C
Glucocorticoids have different degrees of mineralocorticoid activity and stimulate the kidney tubules to retain salt and water (and secrete potassium). Excessive isotonic fluid retention increases the risk of developing hypertension.

19. A
Capillary fragility and decreased strength of the connective tissue predispose to easy bruising. Increased platelet aggregation would reduce a tendency to bruise, and the other answers are not related.

20. D
Glucocorticoids are so named because they stimulate the liver to release glucose into the bloodstream and also reduce glucose uptake by insulin-sensitive tissues such as fat and muscle cells. The combination of increased glucose release and reduced insulin sensitivity predisposes to higher-than-normal blood sugar levels. Cortisol would tend to decrease serum potassium levels, not increase them. The other answers are unrelated.

UNIT XII

CHAPTER 43

Matching

1. c, f, i, d, h, b, e, a, g
2. b, g, e, c, a, d, f
3. b, m, c, l, d, k, a, j, e, i, f, h, g
4. d, a, e, b, c
5. d, b, f, c, a, e
6. B
7. A
8. A
9. B
10. B
11. A
12. B
13. A
14. B
15. A
16. H
17. D
18. E
19. I
20. G
21. F
22. B
23. K
24. M
25. C
26. L
27. N
28. A

True/False

29. T
30. F
31. F
32. T
33. T
34. T
35. T
36. F
37. F
38. T
39. F

40. F
41. T
42. T
43. T

Multiple Choice

44. B
45. D
46. C
47. C
48. B
49. A
50. C
51. C
52. B
53. B

Fill in the Blanks

54. low; fast Na^+ channels
55. Ca^{2+}; glutamate; Mg^{2+}
56. generate action potentials
57. acetylcholine, amine, amino acid, neuropeptide, nucleotide, gases
58. threshold, excitability
59. occipital
60. limbic

CHAPTER 44

Fill in the Blanks

1. 24
2. acceleration-deceleration
3. speech or language
4. birth
5. bacterial; viral
6. hypertension
7. Hemorrhagic; ischemic
8. calcium
9. reperfusion injury
10. Cytotoxic; vasogenic

Multiple Choice

11. B
12. A
13. D

14. B
15. A
16. B
17. B
18. D
19. B
20. C
21. C
22. C
23. C
24. A
25. C
26. B
27. B
28. B
29. A
30. D

CHAPTER 45

Multiple Choice

1. B
2. B
3. D
4. D
5. D
6. B
7. D
8. D
9. B
10. C
11. C
12. B
13. A
14. B
15. D

Fill in the Blanks

16. acetylcholine
17. cerebellum; Parkinson disease
18. sympathetic; blood pressure
19. volume; decrease
20. immune

True/False

21. F
22. F
23. T
24. F
25. T

CHAPTER 46

Matching

1. a, g, c, b, d, e, f, k, j, i, h
2. a, i, b, p, c, j, d, l, e, m, g, k, h, o, f, n

Multiple Choice

3. C
4. B
5. C
6. A
7. B
8. D
9. D
10. B
11. C
12. B

Fill in the Blanks

13. hair; cochlea
14. hypertension; diabetes mellitus
15. Spontaneous or non-traumatic
16. amblyopia
17. myopia; hyperopia; presbyopia
18. cataract
19. age-related macular degeneration (AMD)
20. smoke detector alarms

True/False

21. T
22. T
23. F
24. T
25. F

CHAPTER 47

Matching

1. D
2. E
3. B
4. J
5. L
6. I
7. A
8. C

Multiple Choice

9. B
10. B
11. C

12. D

13. A

14. C

15. D

16. A

Fill in the Blanks

17. opioid; prostaglandin inhibitors (NSAIDs), local anesthetics; heat, cold

18. C

19. psychological or behavioral

20. stimulus transduction, signal transmission, pain perception, pain modulation

UNIT XII: CASE STUDIES

1. C

The lowest possible score on each of the three tests of coma in the Glasgow scale is 1; therefore the lowest possible total score is 3. No response in verbal or eye opening gets a score of 1 each. José has the next-to-lowest motor response and receives a 2 for this indicator, for a total score of 4.

2. C

A Glasgow coma scale rating of 4 is very low (3 being the lowest) and indicates a severe head injury. The motor response indicates that José does not have brain death. Even with a coma score of 3 (no responses), other tests are needed to assess whether the brain is dead.

3. B

The vessels that are located in the arachnoid and subdural space are mostly bridging veins that are susceptible to shear stress and breakage with sudden movements of the head such as those that occur in head trauma. A subdural bleed is usually venous, whereas epidural bleeding is usually arterial, because arteries are located between the skull and dura mater. All of the other choices are arteries and therefore not likely to be the cause of subdural bleeding.

4. A

Measures that reduce the blood volume within the rigid container of the skull would likely reduce intracranial pressure. Mild hyperventilation causes vasoconstriction, and diuretics reduce blood volume, both of which would be expected to reduce blood volume in the cranium. Measures to reduce pain and anxiety would likely reduce cardiac output and blood pressure and also decrease intracranial pressure. Putting the head of the bed down would increase the amount of blood within the cranium because of a change in the effect of gravity on blood delivery to and removal from the head.

5. C

All of the answers are possible consequences of seizures, but an increase in brain metabolism in a brain that is already compromised by ischemia and elevated intracranial pressure would contribute to hypoxic brain damage and is the most important reason for preventing seizure activity in this case.

6. B

These findings are indicative of spinal shock following a traumatic spinal cord injury (SCI). Immediately after SCI and lasting for several weeks, spinal shock is a loss of reflex activity below the level of injury. Profound spinal shock is more likely to occur with a complete transection of the cord than with an incomplete injury. This patient is at risk for autonomic dysreflexia after the spinal shock subsides, but the clinical findings do not indicate it at this time. Recovery from complete SCI is very unlikely.

7. D

The usual signs and symptoms of autonomic dysreflexia include hypertension, bradycardia, pallor below the level of injury, and flushing of the skin above the level of injury. The hypertension can be extreme and causes the symptom of headache and visual changes (such as blurry vision). The high blood pressure triggers the baroreceptor reflex, which reduces the heart rate.

8. B

Signs of weakness on the right side of the body are indicative of a stroke in the left cerebral hemisphere. The language center is in the left hemisphere, and because speech is impaired, this also indicates a left cerebral stroke.

9. A

In the acute phase of stroke, the cardiac and respiratory centers of the brain may suddenly fail, causing the patient to have difficulty maintaining a functional airway, or respiratory muscle control may be impaired. Autonomic instability may also occur. An acute stroke is sometimes said to be a stroke in progress because the loss of function changes quickly over time and the patient must be monitored closely. The other choices are important considerations but are not as important acutely.

10. A
A computed tomography (CT) scan is effective in finding areas of hemorrhage in the brain. This is an important consideration because the acute treatment options are different for hemorrhagic stroke and ischemic stroke. Ischemic stroke includes both embolic and thrombotic causes.

11. A
The patient's history of chronic atrial fibrillation indicates a significant risk for embolic stroke. This occurs because ineffective contraction of the atria allows clots to form in the left atrium, which can become dislodged and travel to the brain. This is such a common problem that patients with atrial fibrillation are anticoagulated to help prevent clot formation.

12. C
A stroke in the left cerebral hemisphere commonly impairs aspects of language processing and speech, called aphasia. All of the other choices are common problems with right cerebral strokes, which affect the sensory and motor function on the left side of the body as well as impair sight in the left visual field.

13. B
L-Dopa therapy is a form of replacement therapy in which a precursor for dopamine synthesis (L-dopa) is supplied to the dwindling number of dopamine-secreting neurons in the basal ganglia. This therapy is effective in reducing symptoms but is not thought to preserve the remaining neurons or promote recovery of neuronal degeneration. As the underlying degeneration of dopamine-secreting neurons continues, L-dopa therapy may become ineffective because it is not effective in its original form and must be processed by the neurons. Because fewer neurons are available, less dopamine is synthesized.

14. C
Although several neuronal abnormalities may occur in Parkinson disease, the loss of dopamine-secreting neurons in the basal ganglia is thought to be responsible for the majority of signs and symptoms. A deficiency of acetylcholine in the cerebral cortex is associated with Alzheimer disease.

15. A
Anticholinergic agents are commonly used in patients with Parkinson disease to reduce symptoms. The neuronal pathways in the basal ganglia that use dopamine are opposed by actions of acetylcholine-secreting neurons, and restoring the balance between dopamine activity and acetylcholine can be helpful. This would involve increasing dopamine activity through L-dopa administration and reducing acetylcholine activity with anticholinergics.

16. D
An improvement in motor activity as evidenced by more frequent spontaneous swallowing indicates an improvement in symptoms. All of the other choices are symptoms of Parkinson disease; if they are becoming more obvious, then a worsening of the disease would be noted.

17. B
The large majority of cases of Parkinson disease are considered to be idiopathic, having no known cause. A few forms of early-onset Parkinson disease have been associated with a genetic abnormality, for example, in the Parkin gene, but an elderly onset is most likely an idiopathic form with no known familial pattern of occurrence.

UNIT XIII

CHAPTER 48

Fill in the Blanks

1. dopamine
2. delusions; hallucinations
3. dysthymia
4. bipolar II; bipolar I
5. delusional disorder
6. glutamate
7. anhedonia
8. seasonal affective disorder

Multiple Choice

9. C
10. C
11. D
12. D
13. A
14. B
15. A
16. A
17. A
18. B
19. C
20. B
21. C
22. B
23. D
24. A
25. B

241

CHAPTER 49

Fill in the Blanks

1. triggers, duration, management
2. physical illness, medications
3. anticipatory, avoidance
4. worry
5. depression, anorexia, Tourette syndrome
6. panic disorder
7. Post-traumatic
8. autonomic instability
9. gradual; years
10. benzodiazepines, antidepressants; β-blockers

Multiple Choice

11. A
12. A
13. B
14. B
15. C
16. B
17. D
18. C
19. A
20. C

UNIT XIII: CASE STUDIES

1. C

Fatigue, weight loss, and insomnia are characteristic manifestations of a depressive disorder. Mania is not present, which would be necessary for a diagnosis of bipolar disorder. There is no anxiety. No disturbances in emotion or aberrant behaviors are described.

2. A

Reduced brain serotonin neurotransmission activity has been hypothesized to be the basic neurobiologic element of depression. Serotonin neurons regulate the activity of many other types of neurons in the brain.

3. D

Benzodiazepines increase the effects of γ-aminobutyric acid (GABA), an inhibitory neurotransmitter in the central nervous system. The result is sedation, reduced anxiety, decreased neuromuscular activity, and amnesia. These would be inappropriate for depression at this point.

4. A

Side effects are likely to present early in treatment, but some of the medications require weeks to be effective. No response now does not mean the drug should be changed and is not indicative of insufficient drug or the need to add another medication.

5. B

Major depression is a chronic illness due to an alteration in the brain's biochemistry and requires long-term management. These drugs have no addictive aspects. Although the dosage may need adjustment, refraining from consuming alcohol does not cure the underlying neuropathologic condition.

6. C

Mania is the hallmark symptom of bipolar disorder. Seasonal affective disorder and dysthymia are depressive illnesses. Schizophrenia is characterized by disordered behavior, thoughts, and feelings.

7. C

Acetylcholine is not implicated at all in bipolar disorder. The depressive mood swing of bipolar disorder is associated with deficiencies of dopamine and serotonin, as they are with major depression. Norepinephrine is a catecholamine, and excess levels are associated with mania.

8. B

Mood stabilization is accomplished with lithium, anticonvulsants, and atypical antipsychotics. Lithium is the most commonly prescribed medication.

9. D

The presentation is characteristic of schizophrenia. Delusions, unusual speech, and disorganized thinking are all positive symptoms, while remaining in one position for prolonged periods is a negative one.

10. A

Individuals with schizophrenia are usually genetically predisposed to the condition.

11. D

Reduced brain volume is a common finding. Sulci enlarge as tissue is diminished. Abnormalities of the cerebellum are not involved in schizophrenia. Decreased nicotinic receptors may be found on autopsy.

12. C

The most common environmental triggers are negative childhood experiences and stress. There is no evidence of abuse as a child, but the pressure of preparing for this important examination is an acutely stressful situation.

13. D

Schizophrenia is a psychotic disorder that should respond to antipsychotic medications that alter dopamine receptor activity in the brain and reduce hallucinations and delusions.

UNIT XIV

CHAPTER 50

Matching

1. d, a, b, c
2. f, a and c, g, h, b, j, i, d and k, e
3. G
4. O
5. U
6. S
7. Q
8. I
9. K
10. F
11. R
12. A
13. E
14. L
15. C
16. N
17. P
18. J
19. T
20. D

Fill in the Blanks

21. calcium; phosphate
22. thyroid hormone, growth hormone, sex hormones
23. size, number
24. released; removed
25. nicotinic
26. lactic acid
27. increase
28. concentric; eccentric
29. cross-bridge
30. striated

CHAPTER 51

True/False

1. T
2. T
3. F
4. T
5. F
6. F
7. T
8. T

9. F
10. T

Fill in the Blanks

11. Greenstick
12. wounds
13. decreased muscle strength
14. rickets; osteomalacia
15. male
16. anticholinesterase
17. actively contracted
18. 3
19. knee
20. D

Multiple Choice

21. A
22. B
23. C
24. C
25. D
26. A
27. B
28. C
29. C
30. D
31. C
32. C
33. B
34. A
35. D

CHAPTER 52

True/False

1. F
2. T
3. T
4. T
5. F
6. T
7. F
8. T
9. T
10. T

Fill in the Blanks

11. calcinosis; Raynaud phenomenon; esophageal hardening (dismotility); sclerodactyly; telangiectasias
12. group A β-hemolytic streptococci
13. unknown
14. Butterfly
15. *Staphylococcus aureus*
16. sacroiliac joints
17. flu
18. ulcerative colitis; Crohn disease

Compare/Contrast

19.

Characteristic	Rheumatoid Arthritis	Osteoarthritis
Systemic manifestations	Yes	No
Inflammatory disease	Yes	No
Symmetric presentation	Yes	No
Pain at rest	Yes	No
Laboratory abnormalities	Yes	No

Multiple Choice

20. D
21. A
22. A
23. C
24. B
25. B
26. D
27. D
28. A
29. C
30. A
31. B
32. D
33. C
34. C
35. A

UNIT XIV: CASE STUDIES

1. B
One of the diagnostic criteria for rheumatoid arthritis is stiffness that lasts at least an hour. None of the other options is significant to the diagnosis.

2. B
Erosion of joints, increasing the joint spaces, is a common finding in rheumatoid arthritis. Decreased bone density and infection are not characteristic of this disease. Rh factor is isolated in the blood.

3. C
The areas most commonly involved in rheumatoid arthritis are the wrists, hands, knees, and feet. If the spine is involved, it is the upper cervical region.

4. A
Flexion contractures are common with advanced rheumatoid arthritis, especially noticeable in the fingers. Pathologic fractures are associated with bone demineralization, which is not a feature of this disease. Pain with rheumatoid arthritis is a common finding from the beginning of the disease process. Tissue elasticity is irrelevant.

5. D
There is a genetic component to rheumatoid arthritis, but the disease is much more common in women than in men.

6. C
Systemic lupus erythematosus (SLE) is an autoimmune disease characterized by type III hypersensitivity, where immune complexes are deposited in the connective tissues.

7. C
As these immune complexes invade the basement membranes of the body's tissues, the resulting inflammatory response progressively reduces their normal functioning.

8. A
Immune complex deposition and the inflammatory process are responsible for these manifestations.

9. B
All of these conditions develop with systemic lupus erythematosus (SLE), but the cardiovascular effects of premature atherosclerosis are responsible for most of the morbidity and mortality.

10. B
Although there is an inflammatory component, osteoarthritis is not considered an inflammatory disease, as is rheumatoid arthritis. All of the other options are associated with rheumatoid arthritis.

11. C

Crepitus in osteoarthritis occurs because of the formation of osteophyte spurs. All of the other options are associated with rheumatoid arthritis.

12. C

Because osteoarthritis is not an inflammatory disease, acetaminophen is very effective for pain relief and anti-inflammatory drugs such as steroids are not indicated. This is a disease of weight-bearing joints, so increased weight bearing will not be beneficial. Isometric muscle exercises are irrelevant to the pain of osteoarthritis.

13. A

Osteophyte spur formation is found only in osteoarthritis. The other options are all part of the pathology of rheumatoid arthritis.

14. D

A fracture near the epiphyseal plate may significantly affect bone growth in children.

15. A

Oblique fractures result from a rotational force along an oblique course (45-degree angle).

16. B

In a compound or open fracture, there is an accompanying wound through which organisms from the environment can gain access to the bone and cause an infection.

17. D

Capillary refill of less than 2 seconds is normal. In compartment syndrome, capillary refill would be prolonged.

18. C

Should the pressure not be rapidly relieved and perfusion restored, the muscle tissue involved will die from ischemia.

19. A

In osteoporosis, the rate of bone resorption exceeds the rate of formation, resulting in porous bone.

20. C

Although chronic glucocorticoid steroid use is a risk factor for osteoporosis, NSAID use is not thought to be associated. All of the other factors are known risks for osteoporosis in women.

21. C

As vertebrae collapse with osteoporosis, significant reduction in height is noted.

22. D

Weight bearing has a major role in maintaining healthy bone and a balance between formation and resorption.

23. C

Weight-bearing activity is effective in preventing osteoporosis in women. Weight loss, although it may be beneficial for other reasons, it is not likely to improve osteoporosis risk. Excessive alcohol intake may increase the risk for osteoporosis.

24. D

Vertebral, hip, and wrist fractures are major complications of osteoporosis.

UNIT XV

CHAPTER 53

Multiple Choice

1. D
2. A
3. B
4. A
5. B
6. A
7. B
8. C
9. A
10. D
11. B
12. A
13. B
14. A
15. C
16. B
17. A
18. C
19. B
20. D
21. C
22. C
23. A
24. D
25. B
26. D

245

27. A
28. B
29. C

Matching

30. D
31. I
32. F
33. E
34. K
35. J
36. H
37. A
38. C
39. A
40. D
41. E
42. F

True/False

43. T
44. F
45. F
46. F
47. T
48. T
49. T
50. T
51. T
52. T

Fill in the Blanks

53. *Candida albicans*
54. Seborrheic dermatitis
55. chancre
56. plants
57. keloid
58. ticks
59. corticosteroids
60. oral mucosa; conjunctiva

CHAPTER 54

Multiple Choice

1. C
2. B
3. C
4. D
5. A
6. C
7. B
8. D
9. B
10. C
11. A
12. C
13. A
14. A
15. B
16. D
17. C
18. D
19. A
20. B

Fill in the Blanks

21. smoke inhalation
22. sebum
23. blood supply
24. third
25. pulse oximetry
26. benzodiazepines
27. 90
28. scald
29. catecholamines
30. hypersecretory
31. debridement
32. electricity
33. 2; 4
34. third
35. 22.5
36. hemoglobin
37. myoglobin; rhabdomyolysis
38. depressed
39. eschar
40. Pressure dressings

1. B

Primary lesions are the original appearance, whereas secondary lesions are those that have been altered, as by scratching. There are no assessment data provided describing the appearance of the rash.

2. A

In children of this age, eczema lesions typically appear on the flexor surfaces of the extremities, especially the antecubital and popliteal areas, the wrists, and the nape of the neck.

3. C

Other interventions include decreasing the frequency of bathing, using tepid water in baths, eliminating alkaline soaps, and using moisturizing creams (especially after baths and washing). Occlusive dressings are inappropriate.

4. B

As a 9-year-old child, B.N should be able to understand that her itchy rash is a kind of allergic reaction.

5. B

When appropriately applied topically, little of the medication is absorbed into the circulation to produce systemic effects.

6. A

As an allergic reaction, systemic antihistamines may be required if more conservative measures cannot control the pruritus. Systemic steroids are avoided; barbiturates are sedative drugs and also inappropriate; antibiotics will not relieve the itching; the condition does not have an infectious cause.

7. C

Retrospective studies have documented that eczema improved in nearly one half of the children as they aged. The predisposition for eczema appears to be inherited, but a specific allergen cannot be identified. Exacerbations and remissions are not features of the condition.

8. B

Superficial partial-thickness burns involve the epidermis to the level of the dermis, and pain sensors remain intact. The most superficial portion of the epidermis is affected in a first-degree burn. If the epidermis, dermis, and subcutaneous tissue are damaged, it is a third-degree burn.

9. B

A burn such as this, covering less than 10% in a child under 10 years of age, is classified as a minor burn injury.

10. B

Scald injuries are best treated initially with cool water, which allows cooling of the scalding liquid as well as the underlying skin.

11. A

A second-degree superficial burn will heal from the perimeter toward the center and will not require grafting, because the dermal tissue remaining is capable of regeneration.

12. D

This type of burn injury typically requires 2 to 3 weeks to fully heal. The blisters will ooze clear fluid, and damaged epidermis will slough. Increased swelling, redness, or purulent drainage from the blisters may indicate a secondary infection.